POWER UP: A YOUNG WOMAN'S GUIDE TO WINNING WITH SPORTS NUTRITION

STEVIE LYN SMITH

WITH
MOLLY HURFORD

STRONG GIRL PUBLISHING

DISCLAIMER: This book is intended for informational and educational purposes only and does not constitute medical, nutrition, or fitness advice. The content is not a substitute for professional guidance from a physician, registered dietitian, or certified fitness professional. Readers should consult a qualified professional before beginning any new training program, making changes to nutrition, or addressing health concerns. The authors and Strong Girl Publishing disclaim any liability for injuries, losses, or damages resulting from the use or application of the information in this book.

All rights reserved. This book or any portion thereof may not be reproduced or used in any manner what- soever without the express written permission of the publisher except for the use of brief quotations in a book review. This publication is designed to provide accurate and authoritative information in regard to the subject matter covered. It is sold with the understanding that neither the author nor the publisher is engaged in rendering legal, investment, accounting or other professional services. While the publisher and author have used their best efforts in preparing this book, they make no representations or warranties with respect to the accuracy or completeness of the contents of this book and specifically disclaim any implied warranties of merchantability or fitness for a particular purpose. No warranty may be created or extended by sales representatives or written sales materials. The advice and strategies contained herein may not be suitable for your situation. You should consult with a professional when appropriate. Neither the publisher nor the author shall be liable for any loss of profit or any other commercial damages, including but not limited to special, incidental, consequential, personal, or other damages.

Text copyright © 2025 by Stevie Lyn Smith / Molly Hurford

Jacket art copyright © 2025 by Strong Girl Publishing

First edition, 2025

Print ISBN 978-1-0688302-9-7

Ebook ISBN 978-1-998743-00-1

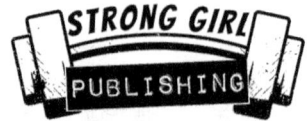

To the young women reading this book, I hope this sparks a shift in how you think about food and your body, not only for sport but to be able to step into your most vibrant and true self.

We aren't here to make ourselves smaller, but to take up space and show the world what we're capable of.

CONTENTS

Foreword   ix
Micha Powell, Olympian and author of Sprinting Through Setbacks

Introduction   xiii

NUTRITION 101   1
1. Macronutrients: What Are They + Why Do They Matter?   2
2. Carbs are Queen   5
3. Protein is a Priority   14
4. Fat is Your Friend   22
5. Micronutrients: What Are They + Why Do They Matter?   28
6. The Performance Plate   39

SPORT SPECIFICS   45
7. Pre-Workout Fueling   46
8. During Training + Competition   53
9. Post-Workout Fueling   63
10. Common Digestive Issues   68

THE IMPORTANT EXTRAS   76
11. Sleep 101   77
12. Understand Your Hormones   81
13. What Happens When You Underfuel?   88
14. What's the Deal with Supplements?   96
15. What Nutrition Trends Get Wrong   104

PUTTING IT ALL TOGETHER   116
16. Eating at Home   117
17. Eating at School   119
18. Eating in the Dorm   123
19. Eating in Your First Apartment   127
20. Grocery Shopping 101   138
21. Simple Recipes for Hungry Athletes   143
22. How to Talk to Experts—And Be Taken Seriously   152
23. Sample Days in the Life   158

24.	Using ChatGPT as a Meal Planning Tool	169
25.	Daily Food Journal Template	174
	Acknowledgements	177
	About the Authors	179
26.	More from Strong Girl Publishing	181
	References	183

FOREWORD

MICHA POWELL, OLYMPIAN AND AUTHOR OF
SPRINTING THROUGH SETBACKS

When I think back on my journey as a professional track sprinter, one of the biggest lessons I've learned is that training isn't just about the hours on the track or in the weight room—it's also about how you fuel your body.

Nutrition has always been a part of my life. I grew up surrounded by the smells and colors of fresh food—my mom and grandmother were my first inspirations in the kitchen. I've always loved cooking and was lucky to be an intuitive eater, making sure my plate was filled with colorful, whole foods.

But like so many young athletes, I didn't always get it right. In college, nerves sometimes got the best of me, and before big races, I'd end up underfueling. My stomach was tight with stress, and I'd try to run on empty.

Eventually, I worked with a dietitian who helped me find simple, easy-to-digest meals—like oatmeal with peanut butter and banana—that gave me both comfort and confidence. That changed *everything*.

Now, my best races are the ones where I've fueled properly before and recovered with protein right after. Fueling became not something to fear, but a key to unlocking my best performances.

I also carried some nutrition myths with me early in my career.

One that stands out was the idea that if I didn't eat within *exactly* 30 minutes of finishing a workout, I'd lose all my progress. That pressure created unnecessary stress—especially as a busy student-athlete.

Over time, I realized that being consistent and intentional matters more than being perfect. A quick protein shake after practice and a hearty dinner later is often enough. The key isn't to panic—it's simply not to skip. And, especially for female athletes, understanding that eating enough (especially when training hard) not only fuels performance but also protects our bodies from injuries and supports long-term development.

That's why registered dietitian Stevie Lyn Smith and Molly Hurford's book *Power Up: A Young Woman's Guide to Winning with Sports Nutrition* is such a powerful tool.

What I love about Stevie's approach is how empowering it feels. Instead of labeling foods as "good" or "bad," she focuses on timing and context. She reminds us that food isn't about restriction—it's about strategy and support. The variety of topics in *Power Up* made this book a true page-turner for me. Digestion issues, complex carbs, sleep cycles, hormones, stress, supplements: it's all here, simplified in a way that feels both relatable and actionable.

Even as a 30-year-old professional athlete, I found myself learning new tools, like how to use the protein formula to optimize my daily intake, which I've already started applying to my own routine.

What makes this book especially important is how it speaks directly to young women. Today, so many athletes are influenced by social media trends: TikTok nutrition hacks, quick fixes, or "one-size-fits-all" advice. But *Power Up* cuts through the noise with science-backed strategies, approachable tips, and even journal prompts that help you connect the dots between your habits, your cycle, your stress levels, and your performance.

That resonated with me deeply, because in my own book, *Sprinting Through Setbacks: An Olympian's Guide to Overcoming Self-Doubt and Imposter Syndrome,* and journal/workbook *Sprinting*

Through Your Setbacks, I encourage young athletes to track, reflect, and celebrate themselves with kindness. Both Stevie's and my message align here: success doesn't come from restriction. It comes from awareness, compassion, and building sustainable habits.

If I could give one piece of advice to every athlete, it's this: fueling looks different for everyone. Find what works for your body, your sport, and your lifestyle. Keep it simple. Use go-to meals and snacks you love. And don't be afraid to ask for help from a professional—you deserve to maximize the effort you're already putting in.

At 30, I can honestly say I've never felt stronger, healthier, or more grounded. That's not just because of training—it's because of how I treat my body through food. The better I fuel, the better I feel, and the more longevity I gain in my sport and my life. So as you open these pages, I encourage you to lean in, take notes, and try things out. This book isn't just about what to eat—it's about how to take care of yourself as a whole athlete and as a young woman stepping into her power. Prioritize your health. Celebrate your body. And remember: every bite you take is an investment in the future you're building.

—Micha Powell
Olympian, Author, and Coach

INTRODUCTION

Dialing in your nutrition—on and off the playing field—isn't easy. But it's a huge part of your success as an athlete. Being properly fueled improves your ability to perform, to recover, and to continue to develop as an athlete. If you're not fueling the work that you're doing, everything becomes harder, even impossible. Understanding the nutrition basics, what a healthy day of fueling the work you're doing looks like, and how different workouts and training days should be fueled is a game-changer for any athlete. And once you have that understanding, developing those good habits does become a lot easier.

Smart nutrition is tricky for everyone, whether you're an athlete or just someone trying to lead a healthier life. First of all, most books written about it tend to start with the assumption that you already know all of the basics. But not only is that unfair—most schools don't teach a lot about nutrition—it is *extremely* unhelpful, because it means that as you're taking in the information, it's without an understanding of those underlying basics. So we're going to start with those and add on from there. Don't feel bad if you're a little unclear about protein, fat and carbohydrates, because to be honest, there's a ridiculous amount of (mis)information out there—and nutrition, especially nutrition for athletes, isn't something that's particularly well-taught in schools, if it's taught at all.

And that's why I wanted to write this book. To demystify nutrition for young women athletes so that you could be equipped to help yourself thrive in sport. I've been in your shoes: Growing up, I was the quintessential team sport athlete. I basically tried all of the sports available, year-round, usually playing on multiple teams at once. There were plenty of double practice days, weekend tournaments, and late nights trying to cram in homework!

In high school and into college, I really honed in on lacrosse, and fell in love with playing goalie. I loved it, but I hit a point towards the end of my freshman year at university where I was a little burned out on competitive team sports and wanted to transfer into a new program of study. I didn't have a lot of options to make both my education and athletic goals align, so I did what a lot of athletes do: I stopped playing lacrosse and I picked up running in my sophomore year after I transferred schools. I ran my first marathon in 2009 and it became the catalyst for getting into all sorts of long-distance endurance sports. I learned to swim and started biking, which led to doing triathlons, which include a swim, a bike and a run. I quickly fell in love with the sport and the challenges it presented. Within my first year of racing, the IronMan—which includes a 2.4 mile swim, 112 mile bike and full marathon—became my goal. I was hooked, so naturally, I did nearly a dozen of them in my twenties. Since then, I've continued to have fun and challenge myself with different events, from long distance open water swim races to an ultramarathon and everything in between. You could say I've found my groove, and an amazing community in endurance sports. But it wasn't a perfect journey. I made a lot of the fueling mistakes that I talk about in this book during that time!

To stay a healthy endurance athlete, having some basic understanding of nutrition is key. Since I was in school to be a dietitian when I started my journey into endurance sports, I had the perks of learning from my own mistakes at the same time I was learning in class. That helped, but even knowing all of the information doesn't always translate into practicing it.

Still, it gave me a major advantage. Combining my passion for being active with my coursework was invaluable to me when it came to staying active in endurance sports. I used it as a driver to take care of myself and my body, and ultimately, to perform well in both training and racing. If I hadn't been my own best guinea pig, fueling my training the way I was learning to teach others to do, I know I would have fallen into a lot of the traps I see young women in now. Even knowing the "right way to fuel" didn't guarantee I actually did it all right! But at least I knew enough to spot early warning signs when things were not going in the right direction. I saw that the young women around me didn't have those same insights and information, and I knew from my own high school and college experience that nutrition was really something you had to be interested in and to learn about on your own time. There weren't a lot of resources available, and the resources that are out there aren't always being shared with young women in ways that are helpful.

A month after racing my first full Ironman in 2012, I officially became a registered dietitian. As I continued racing those longer and longer distances, I naturally gravitated towards a speciality in sports nutrition in my work. It's been fun and a privilege to be able to provide information, guidance, and support to female athletes in a way that I never had in any of my athletic experiences growing up. I want to empower the future generation of young women athletes (you!), and hopefully save you from some costly mistakes on your own journey.

It's hard if you're a young athlete who doesn't have great guidance or support when it comes to nutrition. Especially for high school athletes, coaches are often teachers who love the sport, but may not have a deep well of knowledge when it comes to nutrition for the young female athlete. Then, when you get to college, coaches assume you already know how to fuel and eat well, otherwise you wouldn't have made it this far in your sport. Basically, most young women athletes are on their own, left to—ahem—do their own research. (Not loving that phrase these days, and later, we'll discuss why!) Nowadays, the information coming at you online is, well, a lot. And often inaccurate. And rarely covers the basics of a solid sports nutrition foundation.

That's because a solid sports nutrition foundation and accurate nutrition advice is rarely glamorous. It's usually pretty boring, to be honest. (Sorry in advance.) But stick with it and I promise you'll do a lot better than if you start chugging celery juice every morning and only eating in a two-hour window every day except for all the supplements. (Don't do that. Please.)

This book is packed with all sorts of good stuff. We start by covering some of the basics of every day nutrition, like what the heck protein *actually* is and how much of it you need. We dig into macros and micros, all the buzzy stuff you hear about but may find confusing. It's important to understand what these things are at this basic level so that when trends come at you, you know what the heck people are talking about, and you can make more informed decisions. It also helps you start to understand what a good meal consists of, and where you've maybe missed some key nutrients in the past. And then, we get to the slightly sexier stuff: how you as a young woman athlete have very different needs than the gym bros you see chugging protein drinks on Instagram, or even the 30-year-old fitfluencer who's sharing smoothie recipes on TikTok. Your needs are unique. Not only are we thinking about fueling your performance in training and competition, but we also need to make sure you're fueling your body for normal growth, development and overall good health.

We're here to help you figure out some of the nuances to being a female athlete. If you're between 10 and 25, there's a huge amount of growth that's happening for you during this time,[i,ii] and that means how you fuel now can impact who you are a decade down the line. That's right: How you fuel your training at 15 can make or break your ability to compete at a high level when you're 25.

Finally, we're going to give you the tools and actions that you can take and start to use right away. These are great foundational habits that you will be able to carry throughout your life as an active female. We're going to show you how they actually work in real life, whether you're living at home, in the dorms, or in your first apartment. Heck, we're even going to help you learn to cook a few key meals, how to think about meal planning, and how to navigate the grocery store.

We're here to help you take control, to put your health first *and* be able to show up in your sport and perform at your absolute best.

Throughout this book, we'll get into a lot of nitty-gritty details and explanations of things. But if you only take a few things away from *Power Up*, let it be these key principles: .

- View food through a positive lens. Think about all the great ways food can impact us: it gives us energy, it can be part of our connection with friends and family, and it allows us to feel satisfied, nourished, energized, strong, and like we can perform at our peak!
- Health first, performance second. No matter how high level you are as a young athlete, your health should always be your top priority. Anything that offers short-term performance gains but risks your health isn't worth it.
- As training goes up, eating goes up. Period. You have to fuel your work!
- Get out of the calorie mindset. Ideally, you won't count at all, just learn to visualize food in simple portion sizes when you think about what's on your plate. If you need to pay closer attention to make sure you're eating enough, start to count in grams of proteins, fat and carbohydrates instead of calories. For those who've struggled with diet culture and naturally have that running calorie count, this can be hard to do, but so worth it in the long run.

- Snacks are opportunities. They give you a chance to catch up, to recover better, and to allow your muscles to do their thing.
- Your weight is *not* a performance metric.
- Not everything you eat needs to be for nutrients or performance, joy counts too! Whenever you're debating what to eat, or whether you 'should' eat or not, come back to your Why. Why are you doing this? Is it a restriction you're placing on yourself or are you actually not hungry? Are you not eating the donut because you realize you actually have time to make a sandwich that will be more satisfying, or are you skipping it because you're internally calorie counting?
- It all depends and everyone is unique. If you work with a dietitian or any other medical expert, make sure that they use this phrase at least once every appointment. This is because we are all wildly different and what works for one person may not work for another. Consider this your all-important reminder that you are a unique individual and your nutritional needs are unique as well.

Nutrition can be intimidating. Consider this book your road map to finding your optimal fueling strategies so that you perform at your best both on and off the court. And now, let's get started!

-Stevie Lyn Smith, Registered Dietitian

A quick note: We (Stevie and co-author Molly Hurford, author of the *Shred Girls* series & *Fuel Your Ride*) worked together to bring my (Stevie's) nutrition principles to life in a way that was easy-to-understand for athletes of any age and level. Collectively, we've run the sport gamut from school teams to ultra-endurance events, and we've attempted to include as many sports and common athlete situations as possible in these pages!

NUTRITION 101

IN THIS SECTION, *you'll learn all about the basics of nutrition, the building blocks that will help you better understand the 'why' behind optimized eating strategies, and give you the tools to cut through the nutrition noise.*

1 / MACRONUTRIENTS: WHAT ARE THEY + WHY DO THEY MATTER?

SIMPLY PUT, macronutrients are nutrients your body needs in large quantities to provide energy and also maintain the body's structures and systems so that everything works the way it should. Carbohydrates, protein and fat are macronutrients.

Pretty simple, right?

Well, yes and no. While the macronutrients themselves are pretty basic and you've likely heard of them before, you've also likely heard a lot of misinformation about them over the years. Maybe you heard that fat is bad and should be avoided at all costs. Maybe you've heard that athletes require tons and tons of protein and the other two just don't matter. Maybe you've heard that low-carb is the way to go.

For young women athletes in particular, the short version is that you shouldn't be avoiding any one of these nutrients. They are all necessary and vitally important for your development as an athlete and a healthy human.

When it comes to macros, we like talking about them because shifting to a conversation of protein, fat and carbohydrates is a much more productive conversation than talking about just "calories in, calories out."

For athletes, because of our activity level[i], overall energy needs are higher. And since these three macronutrients provide the energy for our body, we're going to need more of them in general. To break it down—and we'll go into a lot more detail in the next few chapters—carbohydrates are the main sources of fuel for our body and our activities; protein is what allows us to recover, maintain and grow muscle; and fat plays a major role in hormone function, protecting your organs, and meeting our overall energy needs.

But before we get too far along with talking carbs, protein and fat, let's talk about how to keep track of them. While I don't recommend counting anything on a regular or long-term basis, when/if you do need to track food intake, I want you to get in the habit of counting in grams of macronutrients, and forget about calories entirely.

Now, I want to underscore this message: I tend to *not* encourage younger athletes to obsessively track their macros or try to hit certain calorie goals with them—just learn enough about what your usual meals contain so that you can roughly estimate if you're getting enough. We don't need to micromanage, we just need to check in and make sure that what you're eating is falling within total energy and macronutrient percentages that are most beneficial for you.

As a dietitian, when a younger female athlete tells me that she is interested in tracking her macros or counting her calories, I want to know: Why is she interested? Where is this desire to do so coming from? Is it something that she's doing in conjunction with thoughts or beliefs around restriction? Obsessively counting can be one of the early red flags for disordered eating, which can be a huge problem for young athletes.

However, if there's a reason to track intake, like checking in to ensure that you're actually eating enough, counting grams tends to be a better option. That's because unlike calorie counting, which can often feel like a race to the bottom, grams tend to feel a little less triggering, especially if you're someone who has a history of getting a little obsessive about calories.

A lot of us slightly older athletes came up in sport learning to track calories obsessively, and if you ask any woman athlete over the age of 30 how many calories are in a banana and an egg, she will almost certainly tell you it's around 170 total. Calories were *the thing* in the early 2000s and it led to some truly terrible results.

So we don't want you to start memorizing tables of total carbohydrate grams in a banana—around 27, in case you were wondering—but it can be helpful to develop a bit of an internal library of what a serving of carbs, protein or fat looks like in different foods.

Carbohydrates	Fat	Protein
1 bagel = 48 grams	2 tablespoon nut butter = 16 grams	2 eggs = 12 grams
1 medium sweet potato = 27 grams	½ avocado = 12 grams	1 cup cottage cheese = 25 grams
2 handfuls of pretzels = ~30 grams	1 handful of nuts = ~18 grams	2 string cheese sticks = 12 grams
½ cup oats (uncooked) = 27 grams	1 tablespoon olive oil = 14g	1 cup milk = 8 grams
2 fig bars = 38 grams	2 tablespoon flaxseed = 10 grams	1 cup black beans = 15 grams
1 cup orange juice = 26 grams	¼ cup shredded cheese = 9 grams	1 cup Greek yogurt = 17 grams
½ cup rice = ~40 grams	2 whole eggs = 10 grams	1 cup edamame = 17 grams
1 cup dry Cheerios = 21 grams	1 piece salmon = 12 grams	1 piece chicken breast = 27 grams

If you are starting to learn about macros and how much of each is in your meals, using trackers that don't show calories can be helpful—again, calorie count is a number we want to stay away from, unless we're working closely with an expert, someone who is a registered dietitian with a sports nutrition background, like myself. You can also take advantage of AI here and put your meal into ChatGPT or another AI platform and ask for a macronutrient breakdown. It definitely won't be perfect, but it's a good spot to start!

Now, let's dig into each of the macronutrients. The meat and potatoes, if you will. (Sorry in advance for any and all food puns.)

2 / CARBS ARE QUEEN

IN SOME WAYS, carbohydrates; also known as carbs or their scientific abbreviations, CHO; are pretty simple. We need them in order to fuel our training. But they can also be super complicated. Are they good, are they bad, is a vegetable the same as a bagel since they both are in the carb category? It's kind of confusing, since carbohydrates include foods that almost everyone thinks of as "good" like fruit and vegetables, but also the foods that many people assume are bad, like cookies, candy, and soda.

Carbs get split into categories: Simple and complex; sugar, starch and fiber; good and bad, soluble and insoluble fiber, high GI and low GI—and that also adds to the confusion.

In recent years, diets that are low or no carb, even omitting the traditionally "good" ones, have been celebrated. So, what the heck *should* you be eating?

I'll try to keep it simple. The answer begins with why we need carbs, especially as developing athletes. First and foremost, carbohydrates are just plain delicious, and we're big fans of making sure athletes aren't just eating, they're enjoying their food. But more importantly, carbs are the body's primary energy source during the day and especially during exercise, and help us recover as we sleep.

Carbs are converted into glycogen in the body, and glycogen is what allows your muscles to actually perform. With more carbs on board, you can push harder during high intensity workouts while experiencing a lower Rate of Perceived Exertion (RPE)[i].

And it's not just our leg or arm muscles that require carbohydrates: Did you know that our brains also have huge energy demands? We want to make sure that we're meeting the demands for our sport, but also meeting the demands of our brain at school.

When you're eating enough carbohydrates, you'll have more energy, both physically and mentally. Get too little, and you might notice that you're low on energy in practice and you struggle with brain fog and focus in class—and on the playing field when it comes to your ability to work on skills. Being low on carbohydrates in your diet is typically also the reason you start to feel the hunger/anger combination often known as being 'hangry.' Being low on carbs can also tank your mood in a hurry.

Not getting enough carbohydrate has also been shown to potentially disrupt hormonal balance, and can cause you to stop getting your period, even if you are eating enough total calories. It can also impact bone health by potentially decreasing bone density—and unfortunately, that's something you can't easily get back later in life.[ii]

Carbs are also key at a cellular level: They provide the energy for cells, tissues, and organs. They play a role in our blood glucose levels as well as our insulin, cholesterol and triglyceride metabolism. That all sounds pretty intimidating, but don't worry: All you really need to know is that they are incredibly important in order for your body to function at its best.

SIMPLE AND COMPLEX CARBS

The easiest breakdown of carbohydrates is to think about them as simple and complex.

Simple carbohydrates are the ones that are easy to break down in your body, meaning your body has to do less work to turn them into energy. They'll give you that fast burst of energy that helps you sprint to score that goal or catch that fly ball.

Maple syrup, white bread, cookies, cake, sports drinks, gels and bars are all made up of simple sugars, carbohydrates that are already mostly broken down for quick digestion. In sports nutrition terminology, we talk about glucose and fructose as the two types of simple sugars that our muscles primarily use during activity.

Complex carbohydrates are digested slowly and release sugar in the form of glucose into the bloodstream more gradually than simple carbs. They also have more micronutrients in them because they're less processed. This is great for sustained, all day energy, but because it takes more energy and effort for your body to process them, they are less helpful when you eat them around your workouts. Complex carbs include foods like whole wheat and sprouted grains, oatmeal, brown rice, potatoes, cauliflower, fruits and vegetables.

Fiber is a part of complex carbohydrates, and there are two types. Insoluble fiber is the indigestible portion of a plant-derived food—known as roughage—that cannot be completely broken down by human digestive enzymes. Soluble fiber can be broken down by the gut, and when it is, it combines with water to make a gel-like substance in your gut, which helps control blood sugar and allows your body to digest at the right speed.

Fiber helps your body in a number of ways, primarily by moving less-helpful nutrients like too much fat or cholesterol through the body and out in your bowel movements. Fiber is what makes you have good bowel movements (more on that later). It even helps regulate your hormones. We need it, but not too much and not too little.

Fiber is kind of like a Goldilocks and the Three Bears situation: We need our fiber intake to be *just right* so we're having regular bowel movements and naturally detoxifying the body. Take in too little and you're constipated, but eat too much and you'll end up experiencing gut distress or the need to sprint to the bathroom several times during practice.

Examples of Simple Carbs	Examples of Complex Carbs
White bread	Brown rice
White pasta	Whole grain or legume pasta
Crackers	Quinoa
Breakfast cereals	Beans
Juices and sports drinks	Lentils
Fruit chews, energy chews	Oats
Dried fruit	Whole grain bread and bread products
Honey	Starchy vegetables like potatoes
Candy	Vegetables like peppers and asparagus

SERVING SIZE

In general, a serving of carbs is about half to 2/3 of a cup—or a cupped hand—of cooked greens or legumes (beans) or rice. But the serving size that you *should* be eating can be tricky, because what makes sense for a 45-year-old office worker who doesn't exercise regularly and knows they are at risk for type 2 diabetes doesn't make sense for a 16-year-old basketball player.

A great example of this is if we look at bread. Most people assume one slice equals one serving, and that's plenty for a meal. But while that might be true for an adult who isn't trying to fuel for training, for a growing athlete, one slice of bread is never a full serving, because it's not enough to keep you feeling full and keep your muscles working the way that they should. Think two slices, minimum! In fact, for athletes who are training a lot, I want to see three slices on their plate. Even if you're in the offseason or in the middle of a light training week, one slice of bread (unless it's really, really thick) is not enough carbohydrate on your plate.

Usually, the reality is that you're likely not getting enough carbohydrates if you're a serious athlete, so trying to double up on servings at meals or at snack time is a good idea.

A good sign that you are getting enough carbs is feeling like you're fairly level on the physical and mental energy fronts throughout the day. Sure, a hard practice or an exam in algebra may leave you feeling a little drained, but in general, you aren't struggling to concentrate during physics or having to push super-hard to make it through an interval in practice.

Often, it isn't your fault that you're not getting enough carbohydrates, between finding the time to eat, knowing how much to eat, and taking in all the crappy diet culture that young women are bombarded with. It's really hard to know how much is enough with all the crappy info floating around the internet.

Do you know how much carbohydrate you actually need to fuel your training? It's likely a lot more than you think[iii]! For example, a 150 pound (68 kilogram) athlete who is training for a marathon would likely need 6-10 gram per kilogram of body weight per day. This equates to 408-680 grams of carbs per day, the equivalent of 7 to 10 bagels. (Yes, you read that right.)

These carbohydrate targets are evidence-based and intended to promote high carbohydrate availability so that you can train at your greatest capacity[iv]:

Intensity	Carbs
Moderate intensity (~1 hr per day)	5-7 grams of carb per kilogram of athlete weight per day
High intensity (1-3 hrs per day)	6-10 grams of carb per kilogram of athlete weight per day
Very high intensity (~3+ hr per day)	8-12 grams of carb per kilogram of athlete weight per day

To find your weight in kilograms, divide your weight in pounds by 2.2. And remember, a gram of carbohydrate is equal to four calories, so to see how many calories of carbohydrate you need per day, multiply the grams of carbs by four.

WHAT TO KNOW ABOUT ARTIFICIAL SWEETENERS

It's important to know what you're consuming on a daily basis, including how many artificial sweeteners are in your drinks and foods. And it may be more than you think! Often, fat-free foods are sweetened with artificial sweeteners, as are diet sodas, low calorie drinks and seltzers. From more natural low/no-calorie sweeteners like stevia and monk fruit to chemical artificial sweeteners like aspartame and xylitol, there's a wide range of these sweeteners that could be sneaking into your snacks.

While consuming some artificial sweeteners isn't generally a major problem, I recommend steering clear of them for a few reasons. First, because they're a substitute for simple carbohydrate sweeteners like sugar, honey or maple syrup, artificial sweeteners may cause you to eat less carbohydrates/calories overall. This can lead to worse athletic performance and problems with low energy availability. Artificial sweeteners are often added to foods to reduce the calories, which is generally what we're *not* looking to do for athletes. Because our energy needs are so high, we don't need to avoid sugar at all costs.

They're also sneaky. A lot of the time, we don't even realize that we're eating foods that are artificially sweetened, but it's more common than you may realize. They're showing up in low-fat yogurt all the time, but you may not realize that you're getting an artificial sweetener in that snack. Normally, yogurt is a good high-energy snack, but when it has an artificial sweetener, it's actually making it harder for you to meet your energy needs.

Some artificial sweeteners can even cause gut distress for some athletes. There is some research out there on how artificial sweeteners can potentially negatively impact the gut microbiome and gut health (though more research is needed)[v]. You may even notice that eating or drinking foods and beverages with artificial sweeteners can cause gas and bloating.

Additionally, artificial sweeteners are usually significantly sweeter-tasting[vi] than sugar itself. This may cause your taste buds to read sugary foods as less-sweet over time.

Finally, some sweeteners like aspartame are considered unhealthy and possibly carcinogenic (cancer-causing) when consumed in large quantities—as in nine to fourteen cans of diet soda on a daily basis. So it's unlikely that you're consuming that much, but it's important to be aware of if you do use a lot of artificial sweeteners on a regular basis.[vii]

Should you always skip them? Not necessarily, but you should be aware of them. Moderation is key: make sure you're not relying on artificial sweeteners all the time. Pay attention to ingredient lists and see how often you're consuming them. A diet soda or some stevia in an electrolyte drink a few times a week isn't something to worry about, but if your daily yogurt uses stevia leaf extract, consider swapping it to a brand that uses a sweetener like cane sugar, honey or maple syrup so you're getting useful carbohydrates that can fuel your performance instead.

A SAMPLE DAY OF EATING FOR AN ATHLETE

Young athletes, especially female athletes, tend to underestimate the amount of carbohydrate that they need in order to fuel their training, recovery, development and other energy needs. Here's an example of what fueling a high-intensity training day (1-3 hours of training) should look like for a 134-pound (61 kilogram) athlete taking in between 6 and 10 grams (g) of carbs per kilogram (kg) of body weight. This athlete would need between 366–610g carbohydrates for this training day.

(Note: gram totals listed below solely include carbohydrates.)

Breakfast – 110g
    Bagel (60g)
    Peanut butter (4g)
    Honey (20g)
    Orange juice (26g)

. . .

AM Snack – 68g
    Banana (27g)
    Vanilla Greek yogurt (20g)
    Granola (21g)

Lunch – 87g
    Turkey sandwich with lettuce, tomato, onion (30g)
    Pretzels, snack bag (23g)
    Grapes (16g)
    Lemonade (18g)

PM Snack before one hour gym session – 46g
    Granola bar (45g)
    String cheese (1g)

Gym Session – 20g
    Sports drink or fruit juice (20g)

Dinner – 100g
    Burrito: tortilla, rice, ground beef, black beans, toppings (85g)
    Tortilla chips (15g)

Bedtime Snack – 26g
    Pineapple (22g)
    Cottage cheese (4g)

Daily Total: 457g

. . .

If that looked like a lot of carbs, remember that's right in the middle of the targeted amount, not even the high end! This athlete could have eaten even more carbohydrate. If the athlete was doing a longer workout, for instance, they would have needed to add more sports drink or other simple carbs during the workout. So the next time you're worried about eating "too many carbs," don't be. You're almost certainly not.

3 / PROTEIN IS A PRIORITY

WHEN YOU THINK OF PROTEIN, you might think of bodybuilders chugging disgusting-looking shakes, or maybe you picture chowing down on a massive steak after practice. Or maybe you're just confused about what protein is. You've heard of it, you've seen it listed on nutrition labels, you hear influencer-types mentioning it on social media, but honestly, you're just not sure what exactly it is, what it does, why (if) you need it, and if so, how much? We get it. Let's break it down.

Protein is one of the three macronutrients that our bodies need in order to function, and it plays many critical roles in the body. Athletes know that protein is responsible for muscle growth—you can't develop muscle if you aren't eating enough protein. It's also essential for repairing your body after a tough workout. Protein also does most of the work within your cells and is required for the structure, function and regulation of your tissue and organs.

Protein itself is made up of smaller units called amino acids—basically the building blocks of proteins—which are attached to one another in long chains. There are 20 different amino acids that can be combined to make protein, and when all 20 are present in a food, it's considered a complete protein. This matters because if you don't have all of the amino acids, you're not going to have optimal body function.

When you're eating enough protein, you're able to build lean muscle, maintain the muscle you already have, and you'll be better able to recover after workouts. Protein also is vitally important for your hormones to function properly. Some proteins even function *as* hormones: They serve as chemical messengers that regulate different processes in the body, like muscle growth, blood sugar regulation and hydration balance.

Protein is usually broken down into two types: Animal and plant proteins. If you're not following a vegetarian or plant-based diet, you'll find it easier to take in enough protein on a daily basis and get a full range of amino acids. Your protein should still come from a mix of both animal and plant sources, though. And if you are eating plant-based, you'll be able to meet your protein needs, but may need to be a bit more careful and specific about what you're eating.

ANIMAL PROTEIN SOURCES: MEAT, FISH, EGGS, DAIRY

If you're not a following a vegetarian or vegan diet, it's relatively easy to hit your daily protein needs, since most animal products and byproducts are primarily made up of protein, contain the full range of amino acids, and are generally more bioavailable, which means they take less work for your gut to break them down for use throughout the body.

Eggs are often an easy option for young athletes, since they're easy to prepare and are considered a complete protein because they contain all of the essential amino acids we need. And of course, meat options include chicken, turkey, beef, pork, venison or bison. Any fish, from shellfish to salmon, is also a good source.

We are also big fans of dairy as an easy source of protein. Dairy products like yogurt, milk, cheese, and cottage cheese are great options, and Greek yogurt is going to have even more protein per serving. And before you ask: No, yogurt doesn't need to be low or non-fat (see the next chapter about fats!). The full-fat versions are great for athletes who need both the protein and the fat, and are perfectly healthy as long as you don't notice any digestive upset after eating it.

PLANT PROTEIN SOURCES: BEANS, LENTILS, TOFU, NUTS

A lot of people opt to be plant-based for ethical reasons, and if you've chosen to be plant-based because of that, you can still get enough protein. You may also be plant-based in order to eat less saturated fat, if your doctor has recommended that approach to your diet. It will take more effort on your part to get adequate protein, but it's completely do-able.

But if you have chosen to be plant-based, vegan or vegetarian, we do want you to check in on your *'why.'* Why are you plant-based? Is it actually for ethical reasons, or is it a way of restricting what you're eating? It's always a good idea to question your reasons. We absolutely understand why some athletes opt for a plant-based diet for moral or ethical reasons, but we've seen a lot of young women who use a vegan diet as a way to cut calories in a way that seems healthy.

If plant-based eating is your preference, or even if you're a meat-eater who wants to add more plant sources to your diet, there are a lot of options that *do* contain protein. Good plant sources of protein include beans, lentils, chickpeas, edamame, soy milk, pea protein, tofu, tempeh, and nuts.

You can also get protein in some sprouted grain breads—as a plant-based athlete, you'll need to get used to looking at the nutrition labels on foods and scanning for grams of protein. A typical serving of protein should be 20 to 25 grams, so if a piece of bread contains five grams, you would need to eat four pieces to get a full serving of protein.

And this tends to be the difficulty of a plant-based diet, especially for athletes. Because many protein-containing plant-based foods also contain a lot of fiber, you need to eat a larger amount in order to get

20 grams of protein... Plus now you've consumed a significant amount of fiber. While fiber is necessary and healthy, it can lead to some gut distress when consumed close to a workout, so you need to be conscious of it. Fiber also makes you feel full because it's bulky, not because it's calorically dense, which can lead to eating less overall calories by accident. Too much fiber can be very detrimental especially to young female athletes, because your energy needs are so high.

While the plant-based approach is completely fine, as we said, it is important to check in on your motivations for being plant-based, since research[i] has shown that plant-based diets can be used in order to stick to restrictive eating behaviors. (We'll talk more later about restrictive eating, disordered eating and orthorexia.) If you are committed to a plant-based lifestyle, just commit to doing regular protein check-ins to make sure you're getting enough in your diet!

WHAT IS A SERVING OF PROTEIN?

A full serving of protein is about 20 grams of protein. A serving of protein should be roughly the size of your palm, though that tends to only apply to protein-dense solid sources like meat, fish or tofu.

Getting used to what a full serving of protein is can take some work, since women in general tend to underestimate serving sizes—the amount of yogurt that you need to eat to get that 20 grams of protein may surprise you! For foods that aren't as easy to eyeball, check the serving size on the nutrition facts, and make sure that you're actually eating that amount. For example, a serving of Greek yogurt is one cup, which may be much more yogurt than you're used to scooping out. If you're trying to dial in your protein consumption, a food scale or measuring cups may be a good way to figure out what that serving of yogurt should look like.

You don't need to be precise every time, but having a sense of what 20 grams of protein from Greek yogurt or tofu looks like is a helpful skill. It's not about counting calories, it's about gaining confidence in understanding how much protein you're taking in. You may be surprised at how badly you've been underestimating serving sizes!

A few of our fave protein sources:

	Serving Size	Grams of Protein
Salmon	4 oz	23
Tuna (can or pouch)	3oz can	16
Egg	2	14
Tofu	½ cup	10
Greek yogurt	1 single serve container or 1 cup	17
Cottage cheese	1 cup	28
Turkey	3 oz	24
Chicken	3 oz	27
Beef	3 oz	25
Lentils	½ cup cooked	9
Edamame	1 cup cooked	17
Black beans	½ cup cooked	8

WHAT ABOUT PROTEIN POWDER?

A lot of athletes assume that protein powder is a good thing. And it can be an important tool in your dietary toolbox! But while protein powder can be a useful supplement, I prefer that athletes aren't relying on it. Instead, most of the time, you should be getting your protein from food. When you eat whole foods, you're also getting a lot of other micronutrients (nutrients you need in small quantities, like vitamins and minerals). And there is a lot of research showing the positive effects of eating the actual macronutrients and micronutrients together[ii] in real foods instead of taking a handful of supplements along with your protein shake.

If you're often in a rush between practices and you're trying to add more protein to your diet, a pint of simple chocolate milk will provide nearly the same amount of protein as a scoop of protein powder, and it also contains other essential vitamins and minerals, as well as carbohydrates that are essential to your recovery post-workout... Plus it's cheaper and infinitely more delicious. (It's also easy to find in the dining hall or any convenience store!)

If you are going to use a protein powder—because yes, they are convenient and can be helpful for busy athletes!—look for one that has been third-party tested and has an NSF Certified for Sport or Informed Sport designation, which means that it has been tested and doesn't contain any substances banned by the World Anti-Doping Agency, something that's vitally important for athletes who are competing in any collegiate or professional sport. Because supplements are largely unregulated, they can contain banned substances (purposefully or accidentally due to cross-contamination) and can also contain ingredients not listed on the label. For instance, one study found that 40 percent of the 133 protein powder products they tested had elevated levels of heavy metals.[iii]

HOW MUCH PROTEIN DO YOU NEED?

The recommendation for athletes is to have 1.4 to 1.7 grams of protein per kilogram of body weight per day[iv]. Aim for 1.7 grams per kilogram during harder training weeks, and drop down to 1.4 grams per kilogram when your load is lighter.

Confused? To find out your protein intake, take your bodyweight in pounds and divide it by 2.2 to get your weight in kilograms, then multiply by 1.4 and 1.7 to find your protein range.

Here are a few examples:

Body weight (pounds)	Grams of protein per day
110	70-85
125	80-97
140	89-108
155	99-120
170	108-131
200	127-155

For a 140-pound athlete (63.5kg) with a recommended intake of 89 to 108 grams of protein per day, this could break down to three meals with 25 grams of protein each, plus two snacks with 5 to 10 grams of protein in each for a lighter training week, or three meals with 30 grams of protein each plus two snacks with around 10 grams of protein in each for a heavier training week.

If you're eating three meals a day and a pre- and post-workout snack, you should be able to get enough protein pretty easily. It becomes more difficult if you're skipping meals or snacks—which we never recommend for athletes. If you don't have time to eat a real meal throughout the day, make sure that you're getting enough protein at the meals you are making time for and work on adding more easy snacks throughout the day.

While technically, there's no upper limit on protein consumption, there is a point where it's simply not doing you any good, because your body can only use so much of it at a time[v]. However, it's hard to hit the point of overconsumption unless you're primarily eating chicken breasts for every meal, and in bulk. You may notice some gut issues if you go too hard on the protein, and may struggle with some constipation and cramping, but otherwise, you likely won't experience any major problems. It just won't be useful. (On the flip side, eating more and more protein also won't cause you to develop Popeye-style muscles, so don't stress about putting on 'too much muscle' if you increase your protein.)

HOW DO YOU KNOW YOU'RE NOT GETTING ENOUGH PROTEIN?

Basically, everything falls apart if you're not getting enough protein. You're going to lose muscle mass, which is going to impact your strength and your performance. You can also have feelings of weakness and fatigue. You may start to notice that you're sluggish and you experience brain fog—that feeling where you struggle to focus or just think clearly. You may experience sleep disruptions. Your nails and hair may seem more brittle. You may notice that after workouts, you feel under-recovered, have a lot of muscle soreness and tightness, and just can't get on top of feeling *good*. Injuries won't heal quickly, and you may get sick more often. If you get bloodwork done, you may have an iron deficiency[vi].

If you're worried you're not getting enough protein, track your intake for a few days or a couple of weeks. You can do it by hand, listing everything out in a note app on your phone (and even asking ChatGPT or another AI tool to tally up grams of protein in your meals—it won't always get it perfect, but it's usually pretty close!) There are also apps like Cronometer that allow you to track macronutrients without counting calories if you toggle the settings to turn off the calorie count. This can be helpful if you find that calorie counting apps trigger you. Finally, you can also work with a dietitian, preferably one who specializes in sports nutrition, who will take a handwritten food diary and assess it for you if recording your food in an app is too triggering.

4 / FAT IS YOUR FRIEND

LET's start with the most important point: Eating something that contains fat doesn't mean it gets stored in your body as fat, or that it will make you gain weight. In fact, fat is a necessary macronutrient[i] that is key to providing energy. It lets your body access certain vitamins that can only be processed with certain types of fats, and produces hormones that are absolutely vital for women of all ages. So yes: You need fat.

Like we said about carbs: Any diet that tells you to cut out a macronutrient group isn't going to be a diet that will serve you as an athlete or as a young woman who's still developing hormonally. (More on that later!)

The body uses fat for energy storage, cell membrane building, fighting inflammation, hormone production, and processing certain vitamins like vitamins A, D, E and K[ii]. The hormone production aspect in particular is key for female athletes: If we don't get enough fat, we aren't able to produce hormones like estrogen or progesterone properly, and that can have seriously negative effects on both our health and our athletic careers[iii]. These hormones impact female physiology: our growth, menstrual function (your period), bone health, and overall well-being. And protein and carbs *can't* do these things, which means you need to be eating enough fats, ideally from a wide variety of sources. There's no replacement for fats.

Fats themselves are made up of fatty acids and there are a few different types: monounsaturated and polyunsaturated fats, saturated fats, and trans fats. The two types of unsaturated fat are typically considered the healthy types of fats, while saturated fat sits somewhere in the middle. Then, and here's where it does get into 'fat is bad' territory, there are trans fats, which are mostly a byproduct of the industrial processing of oils. Trans fats are actually banned in most countries due to how unhealthy they are.[iv] Trans fats used to be incredibly common in things like baked goods and animal/dairy product substitutes like margarine, and they're a big reason that fat got a bad rap a couple decades ago! Luckily, they're mostly a non-issue now since most countries have banned the use of them in food.

How can you tell which fat is which? Mono- and polyunsaturated fats (sometimes called MUFAs and PUFAs, which sounds hilarious) are typically liquid at room temperature and include things like olive oil, while saturated tend to be solid when at room temperature—like butter. MUFAs and PUFAs are more commonly found in plant-based fats and seafood, while saturated fats tend to come from animal sources, like full fat dairy. MUFAs and PUFAs are generally accepted as healthy fats, while saturated fats are more of a mixed bag.

- **Monounsaturated fats (MUFA):** Olive oil, avocado, most nuts and seeds
- **Polyunsaturated fats (PUFA):** These Omega-3 and Omega-6 fats include salmon and other fatty fish (tuna, mackerel, trout, herring), ground flax and flaxseed oil, walnuts, hemp hearts, chia seeds
- **Saturated fats:** Beef, lamb, pork, poultry, lard, tallow, butter, cheese, ice cream, coconut, palm oil, palm kernel oil, some baked/fried foods, full fat dairy

Eating a wide variety of MUFAs and PUFAs is important, especially since these unsaturated fats are anti-inflammatory and are typically found in foods that contain other key micronutrients as well. Saturated fats are much easier to come by if you eat a "standard American diet" that includes dairy and red meat, so you generally don't need to worry about actively including them in your daily intake—just don't avoid them, and you'll likely get enough.

Usually, we don't have to intentionally work too hard to get fat at our meals, because it's usually going to be contained in something that's already on our plate, whether it's the oil that our vegetables were stir fried in or if we're having some eggs or salmon as protein, since those animal products contain fat as well.

That's why it's important to consider the whole food when thinking about your food choices, particularly when it comes to saturated fat, and try to optimize your selections accordingly. For example, a hamburger and a donut may have similar grams of saturated fat, but with beef, you're also getting a lot of micronutrients like iron versus the lack of micronutrients you'd get in a fried donut with a similar amount of saturated fat. (However, if you're really craving a donut, we'd never say you should avoid them entirely!)

There is such a thing as too much fat in your diet, or at least, too much fat that isn't doing your body any good. While we don't believe in avoiding any foods entirely, avoid fried foods as much as possible, since those tend to be fried in less-healthy oils and contain minimal additional vitamins and minerals, if any. If you realize that you're eating donuts for breakfast, french fries with lunch, and fried chicken for dinner, that's a sign that you need to shift away from the fried foods for at least one or two meals per day.

That doesn't necessarily mean you need to eat less calories, by the way! It just means you should be prioritizing healthier options like an extra serving of sweet potatoes, sautéed vegetables and grilled chicken over that single piece of fried chicken that leaves you feeling stuffed. Often, the issue with fried foods is that they make you feel full (and sometimes a little bit sick) and that means you end up skipping the foods that are helping your body repair and recover.

What we really don't want you to do is get freaked out about certain types of fat. Every few years, there are shifts in the trends around what fats are 'good' and which fats are 'bad' and even which fats are 'superfoods' that you should be drinking on a daily basis. The simple thing you need to know about fat is to ignore the noise around any single type of fat and instead, focus on getting your fat from a wide range of sources. There is no reason to take shots of any type of oil on a daily basis. Ignore the trends, stick to the basics.

Usually people who don't get enough fats in their diet are intentionally trying to avoid it or trying to cut calories. But fats should make up at least roughly 25 percent of your overall intake,[v] which doesn't take much since a gram of fat is denser than carbs or protein and contains 9 calories. (By comparison, a gram of carbohydrate or protein are 4 calories each).

A healthy day of eating an appropriate amount of fat could look like a tablespoon of olive oil to sauté two eggs for breakfast, a cup of Greek yogurt with a spoonful of mixed nuts at lunch, and a salmon filet sautéed in olive oil for dinner with a scoop of ice cream for dessert.

That also means *stop it* with the 'balsamic vinegar only' salad dressing and no-fat options. We call this the No Sad Salads Rule and we cannot stress it enough. You do not need to use a no-calorie salad dressing, especially as an active athlete. You also don't need the non-fat Greek yogurt. We see this all the time, especially with women. Many of us were raised hearing that fat was bad, or that low calorie options are the "right" options for women. Not true at all. In fact, this is complete and total crap! But it's a hard habit to break if you've been buying the non-fat option or opting for the fat-free salad dressing for years.

The only caveat here is that you do need to be careful with foods that are high in fat around exercise. Unlike simple carbs, which are rocket fuel for your muscles pre- and in-workout, fat isn't going to be helpful in your training. It slows down digestion, so we want to limit our intake immediately before or during exercise. (That said, if you love a peanut butter and jelly bagel pre-workout and your stomach doesn't bother you during training, that's fine—people respond differently to fat. For some people, even that teaspoon of peanut butter makes them feel bloated and uncomfortable, for others, it feels completely fine.)

If you're not sure if you're getting enough fat, ask yourself: *How do you feel after your meals?* If you feel satiated (meaning comfortably full) for at least a couple hours after meals, that's a good sign. Often, if you're avoiding fat, you feel hungry again after meals quickly. You can also ask yourself: *Can you spot the fat on your plate?* Again, sometimes it's hiding since you've sautéed veggies in oil, have a piece of salmon, are eating a parfait with full-fat yogurt with a sprinkle of nuts and seeds on top, or put an oil-and-vinegar dressing on a salad. Start to practice spotting the fat on your plate at each meal and make sure you can point it out. If you can't, you may not be eating enough.

However, while you do need enough fats in your diet, you almost certainly don't need to be supplementing with fancy fat-based supplements that are marketed to athletes—we'd rather see you getting your fats from actual food. It's tastier and more satisfying that way! Things like Omega-3 fatty acids and fish oil in capsule form are often sold as wellness-based supplements, but it's better to get your fat from actual food sources when possible. In the dining hall or grocery store, look for foods like salmon, flax, chia, avocado, and walnuts that are high in Omega-3s[vi]. Nuts and seeds are often the easiest for athletes who are new to cooking and eating healthy, since they can be mixed into cereal or a yogurt bowl or smoothie or salad, and provide a wide range of vitamins and minerals in addition to healthy fats.

If you've been skimping on fat for a long time, you may notice more injuries and bouts of illness, and an inability to recover quickly. You may also notice brittle hair or nails, or dry skin. Finally, a loss of your period may indicate you're not eating enough fat to produce the hormones your body needs[vii]. This is in part due to the lack of energy, but can also be caused by your inability to process vitamins A, D, E and K, which are important for the recovery processes. Often, athletes get bloodwork done and find that they have low vitamin D levels and they start to supplement with Vitamin D capsules in order to solve the problem… but if you don't have enough fat in your diet, the Vitamin D you're taking won't be processed—it'll just end up excreted in your urine.

Don't beat yourself up if you're reading this and realizing, 'Oh no, this is me!' This isn't your fault, this is a society-level problem because of how we were taught to always go for the low- or no-fat option. But now that you know just how important fat is, make the switch to the regular salad dressing (or make your own with olive oil, balsamic vinegar, maple syrup and whole grain mustard—delicious!). Opt for the full-fat or—at a minimum—the low-fat yogurt instead of nonfat. Don't be scared: You'll likely notice that you actually stay fuller feeling for longer after meals, and may even see some positive aesthetic side effects like better skin, hair and nails thanks to your newfound ability to process vitamins. And with your body in better hormone balance thanks to appropriate fat intake, you'll experience better sleep, more sustained energy, and possibly even a better overall mood!

5 / MICRONUTRIENTS: WHAT ARE THEY + WHY DO THEY MATTER?

Ahh, micronutrients. The little guys, if you will. If macronutrients are the big rocks in a jar, micronutrients are the pebbles and sand that fill in the gaps around those rocks. Simply put, micronutrients are the vitamins, minerals and electrolytes that we need to keep our system functioning optimally.

Here, we're looking at the important ones for young women athletes to be aware of, but there are dozens more that are vital to bodily functions—and that can cause serious issues if you're in a deficit. Luckily, most people can get the micronutrients they need simply by eating a well-rounded, varied diet and making sure that they're not just eating the "right" foods, but are eating enough overall.

VITAMIN D

Why is Vitamin D important for athletes?

Vitamin D supports muscle contraction and reduces inflammation, helping you recover faster after intense training sessions and races[i]. It also aids in calcium absorption, which helps keep your bones strong–and stronger bones mean less risk of stress fractures and other bone-related injuries!

Logging long training hours can weaken immunity, leaving you susceptible to illness. But Vitamin D supports immune system function so you can stay healthy and consistent in your training. And finally, as an athlete, your heart does a lot of work. Vitamin D plays a role in maintaining heart health and supporting efficient oxygen delivery to muscles.

How do I get Vitamin D?

Sunlight! Just 10-30 minutes of midday sun exposure a few times a week can help your skin produce Vitamin D[ii]—but in winter, that's often not enough since the sun's rays aren't as direct, especially if you live in a northern area or don't get outside when it's light out.

Food sources rich in Vitamin D include fatty fish (salmon, mackerel, sardines), egg yolks, fortified foods like milk, cereals, and plant-based alternatives and, weird as it may sound, mushrooms that are exposed to sunlight.

Sometimes, diet and sunlight aren't enough—especially if you live above the 37th parallel (anywhere north of San Francisco, which covers a lot of ground in North America!). Shorter days and weaker sun rays mean your body produces less Vitamin D during winter, making it even more important to focus on getting enough of this vital nutrient. But check with your doctor or a dietitian before supplementing, and always look for the NSF Certified for Sport label or similar third party certification.

How do I know I'm getting enough Vitamin D?

Not sure if you're getting enough Vitamin D? If you're getting sick or injured often, this is worth taking a closer look at. To see if you need more vitamin D, you will want to ask your doctor for a simple blood test to check your levels. (But as we mentioned in the last chapter, to absorb the Vitamin D you are taking in, you do need to be getting enough fat in your diet!)

IRON

Iron is more complicated than what you may have heard, which—if anything—was likely just "young women need more iron and need to supplement to get it." That's because like Vitamin D, it's a micronutrient that's necessary, but can be hard to get from food alone.

Iron is an essential component of hemoglobin (blood), and one of its main purposes is to transfer oxygen from the lungs to the tissues. Iron also helps produce adenosine triphosphate (ATP), which is essentially the fancy way to say it helps kickstart our body's energy systems[iii]. It also plays a role in immune function. Because of this, low iron levels can lead to fatigue, poor performance, increased chance of illness, and slow recovery.

Most of your body's iron is recycled to be used again and again. That's why athletes, especially girls and women[iv,v], tend to end up with low iron levels. Your body is breaking down old red blood cells to reuse their iron for new hemoglobin production. But as an athlete, you're also breaking cells down with high-impact training like running. Added to that, women also lose red blood cells during menstruation. If you have a lot of cell turnover, you're putting a lot of stress on the system.

That's why we need to make sure we're taking enough in. Ideally, you're getting your iron from different types of food sources. And here's where it gets a little tricky. There are two types, heme and non-heme iron. Heme iron tends to be animal-based and is more readily available and better used by the body, while non-heme iron comes from vegetarian sources and requires more work to process.

Iron is a mineral that is naturally found in many foods, and is also added or fortified into many food products. You also can get it in the supplement form—but that's not always a good idea!

Heme iron-rich foods include lean red meat, poultry, fish, organ meats like liver, and shellfish.

Non-heme iron-rich foods include plant-based sources like

lentils, beans, tofu, spinach, and fortified iron products like breads, bagels and cereals.

To maximize absorption, pair iron sources with foods containing Vitamin C, like citrus fruits, to help boost absorption. Avoid consuming calcium rich foods like dairy, kale, tofu and any calcium-fortified foods as well as coffee or tea when eating iron-rich meals, as those things can inhibit or block absorption.

You don't need every meal to be a double burger in order to get enough iron: A single burger made with lean red meat and a cup of spinach in a day along with an overall healthy diet would provide plenty of iron.

Young women athletes tend to be at risk for low iron levels for a few reasons[vi], so before you stress about your exact iron numbers, look at the basics:

- Are you eating enough in general? Low carbohydrate intake can negatively impact iron status, even though most carb-rich foods aren't high in iron. Often, athletes who have low iron are underfueling overall, and in these cases, supplementing with iron won't solve the problems that they're having.
- Are you including iron-rich foods in your diet regularly? (If you are choosing to not eat animal products and meat, this is going to be harder, but it's not impossible! You just need to be more aware of the amount of iron you are getting in your food.)
- Are you getting enough rest and recovery? If you're not, no amount of iron supplementation will make your body start to process it properly.
- Is your digestion decent? Overall body inflammation and chronic GI (digestive) issues can lead to lower iron stores.
- Physical symptoms can include cold hands and feet, pale skin, shortness of breath, rapid heartbeat, headache,

dizziness, confusion, and in some cases, brittle nails, hair loss, sleep disruption and Restless Leg Syndrome (twitching legs at night). You'll also feel fatigued and find it hard to recover from training.

If you're noticing any of these symptoms, ask your doctor to test your iron levels—but ask for a full iron panel plus ferritin, because a basic iron test won't tell you the whole story.

If you're considering a supplement, ask your doctor or dietitian for a recommendation specific to your needs. There are so many types of iron available at the pharmacy in the supplement aisle, and they aren't created equal! (In fact, often these supplements are far too high in iron and can actually end up elevating your iron to a toxic level—which can cause digestion issues and ironically may also cause symptoms similar to low iron![vii])

And if you are prescribed an iron supplement due to low iron, think of it as a Bandaid, not a solution. You shouldn't be relying on iron supplements for the long term, because you need to address the actual issue of *why* your iron is low. Yes, an iron supplement can be helpful—but more importantly, you need to understand why you need it in the first place, because there may be better ways you can be supporting your body and your training.

CALCIUM

Athletes demand a lot from their bodies, and calcium is one mineral that keeps everything running smoothly—far beyond just building strong bones. Especially in weight-bearing activities like running, you're putting a repetitive stress on your bones. Calcium is essential for maintaining bone density and preventing stress fractures—unfortunately a common injury in endurance athletes. For female athletes, this is even more critical, as hormonal fluctuations can impact bone health[viii].

Calcium also plays a direct role in muscle function. When you exercise, calcium is released to help muscles contract. Afterward, it's reabsorbed to allow muscles to relax. And remember, your heart is a muscle, and calcium is vital for keeping it beating steadily. It helps regulate your heart rhythm during long training sessions, ensuring consistent blood flow to your muscles and organs.

Calcium supports the activation of enzymes involved in breaking down glycogen (your body's stored form of energy). This ensures your muscles have the fuel they need for sustained activity during training or competition. Post-workout, calcium helps in tissue repair and adaptation to training. It also plays a role in minimizing inflammation, which helps speed up recovery time between sessions.

Finally, Relative Energy Deficiency in Sport (REDs) is a condition involving low energy availability, leading to dysfunction of several body systems, bone loss, and menstrual dysfunction in females.[ix,x,xi] Prioritizing calcium, alongside proper fueling, helps support bone health and overall performance.

Low calcium levels can lead to muscle spasms, impaired nerve signaling, and reduced endurance capacity. If your calcium levels are low, your muscles may feel weak, fatigued, or cramping as though they're being squeezed in a vice even though you didn't do an intense workout to cause that feeling.

Athletes are at higher risk of having low calcium because we sweat out calcium[xii]. Aim for at least 1,500 mg of calcium per day[xiii] by consuming calcium-rich foods, like dairy products, fortified plant-based milks, leafy greens, broccoli, almonds, tofu, or sardines. Pair calcium-rich foods (like milk or spinach) with Vitamin D sources for optimal absorption.

Timing matters: Make sure you're getting calcium in different foods throughout the day, not just in one meal. If you're working on improving your iron levels, it's important to avoid eating iron and calcium rich foods together—calcium can compete with iron for absorption in our gut when we eat them together.

MAGNESIUM

Magnesium is an electrolyte and it's also an essential mineral. We tend to think of it as being important for sleep or for avoiding cramping during sport[xiv], but it does a lot more than that. It plays a critical role in over 300 important cellular reactions, primarily around energy metabolism, cell growth, and protein synthesis. It helps maintain normal nerve and muscle function, including not just those quads and hamstrings, but also your heart. It impacts your immune system and bone health. Magnesium really does do *a lot*.

Good news: Like iron, it's easy to get enough magnesium from an overall healthy diet. It's not hard to find it in foods: nuts and seeds, especially pumpkin seeds, are great sources. Peanut butter, avocado, baked potatoes, brown rice, yogurt, salmon, dark chocolate, milk and soy milk are all great sources. Many electrolyte drinks will also include a small amount of magnesium, though ideally, you're getting it mostly from food instead of from powders or tablets.

Similar to iron, the best way to make sure you're getting enough magnesium is to make sure that you're eating enough overall, and that your diet is varied and contains at least a few of the foods listed above.

If you have a long-term magnesium deficiency, it can lead to bone stress reactions and stress fractures. If you're not getting enough magnesium, you may also notice that you experience more sleep disruptions, even Restless Leg Syndrome (twitching legs at night). You may even notice some cramping during your training, though that can also be caused by low amounts of other key electrolytes like sodium, so it's not a reliable indicator of low magnesium.

VITAMIN B12

B12 deficiency[xv] is a common micronutrient deficiency in many parts of the world, but it doesn't get the same amount of press that Iron or

Vitamin D do when it comes to athlete health. However, B12 helps make DNA—your body's mapping tool—for all of your cells, so it's pretty important. It also helps keep your body's blood and nerve cells healthy. B12 is a water-soluble vitamin that is often added to foods to fortify them—so if you're in North America and eating a pretty well-rounded diet and getting enough calories overall, it's usually not something to worry about. But if you're underfueling, it can become a problem.

B12 is found in a variety of animal foods, but plant foods have no B12 unless they're fortified with it, so vegans and vegetarians need to be aware of making sure they're opting for foods that are fortified[xvi]. Fish, meat, especially liver, poultry, eggs, dairy products, clams, and oysters are the best choices. Breakfast cereals that are fortified in B12 as well as nutritional yeast are options for plant-based athletes. (Nutritional yeast is also tasty sprinkled on popcorn!)

Your body naturally stores 1000 to 2000 times as much B12 as you typically eat in a day, so the symptoms of B12 deficiencies can take several years to appear. You may feel tired or weak, have pale skin, heart palpitations (feeling like your heart is fluttering or skipping beats), tingling in hands and feet, loss of appetite, soreness in your mouth and tongue and unexplained weight loss.

B12 deficiency can also result in megaloblastic anemia, which is a condition similar to anemia—low iron—where people can feel tired and weak. Because of that, sometimes it can be confused with iron deficiency. You can also end up with a deficiency regardless of your diet simply depending on your genetics[xvii], so if you are noticing those feelings of being tired and weak and you're not anemic and you are eating enough, consider asking your doctor to check your B12 levels to rule out a deficiency.

SODIUM

Sodium—AKA salt—is important beyond your performance in your sport, though you mainly will hear about it as a vital electrolyte you need to take in to replace the sodium that comes out when you sweat. But sodium controls so much in the body! It's important for stress response, balancing fluids and pH, and regulating blood pressure. It impacts your stomach acid, which can affect digestion. It plays a role in nervous system function, muscle function, and insulin sensitivity[xviii].

"Salty foods" is the obvious answer here, along with electrolyte drinks. Athletes need to be aware of their intake and pay attention to their sodium consumption—especially athletes who are plant-forward and who tend towards whole foods even in training. Some athletes tend to eat fewer packaged and processed foods, which means they're getting a lot less sodium than the average American[xix]. While we recommend eating lots of fruits, vegetables and simple meals like chicken and rice, if you're someone who avoids sauces and seasonings to keep your calories lower, you're likely missing some of the sodium your body needs, unless you're also adding electrolytes to your water.

Most of us are able to get enough sodium simply by salting our food and/or intentionally including salty snacks like pretzels and pickles. So before you start chugging pricey electrolyte drinks, I would start with asking: "Am I eating enough? Can I salt my foods? Can I add salty snacks to my routine? Am I making sure I'm having some sports drink before and after practice?" If you're doing that, you likely don't need to supplement with electrolyte tabs the rest of the day.

If you're using electrolyte drinks during practice, make sure they have at least a small amount of carbohydrates in them as well. If you don't have carbs with your sodium, it's harder for the body to actually use that sodium[xx].

In a worst case scenario, you may end up with hyponatremia if your sodium levels get too low during sport. Symptoms of hyponatremia[xxi] in exercise include headache, fatigue, nausea, vomiting, muscle cramps, confusion and seizures. And it can be fatal.

There is a fine line, though: Take in too much sodium and you'll feel increased thirst and potentially experience bloating, swelling in your hands, feet and face, headaches, nausea, fatigue, and frequent urination. In severe cases, too much sodium can cause confusion and seizures. More is not always better! We want to find just the right amount for you.

If you're losing more sodium through your sweat than you're replacing in your drinks and food, you may notice digestion issues, cramping and a decrease in performance[xxii]. You may tend to perform worse in the heat. And if you see noticeable white salt grit on your clothing and skin, this is a sign that you're a salty sweater. Salty sweaters may need two to four times of the daily recommended sodium intake to replace what they lose while training!

Sweat rate testing is one of the best ways to check that you're adding enough sodium to your water bottles and in-training snacks so that you're staying on top of those losses. Sodium and chloride are the electrolytes that are lost in the highest quantities in our sweat, and the ones that most impact our performance outcomes. We'll talk about sweat testing later in this book, but the short version is that you need to make sure that as you sweat out sodium, you're replacing it. If you aren't getting enough sodium, you'll notice.

The good news is that low sodium is often an acute problem, meaning it's only happening during a sweaty practice and then you bounce back. It's much less common for your sodium to stay low, unless there are other issues at play. I have seen some athletes who have eating disorders or disordered eating who develop chronic low sodium hyponatremia, which is persistently low sodium levels. This tends to be caused by food restriction, which means less opportunities to take in sodium, and excessive fluid intake—too much plain water—in addition to hormone imbalances brought on by overall restriction.

It's about finding a balance: If you feel like you are a very salty sweater and you really struggle to stay hydrated, if you're really struggling with cramps and some of those feelings of dehydration like having a headache after practice, that can be a very good sign that you are not hitting the mark with hydration. Reaching out to a sports dietitian to do some sweat testing and making an individualized plan can make a big difference to your performance.

6 / THE PERFORMANCE PLATE

WHILE EVERY MEAL should include every macronutrient—carbs, proteins and fats—there are tweaks you can make depending on what you're doing or have just done. Most of the tweaking that happens is related to the carbohydrates that are on your plate, but your fat and protein will adjust slightly as a result.

Rather than saying every meal should have an exact number of carbs or grams of protein and fat, we like to think about setting up our meals as plates based on training intensity levels. These plates show how your food looks on a plate (roughly) based on the amount of activity you're doing that day or have already done. Note that these aren't just your pre-workout meals, this is how *every* plate should look throughout the day.

Every meal (with the exception of right before training or during training) ideally includes a combination of carbohydrate, protein and fat.

As you'll see, the types of carbs you need in each meal will vary depending on your activity level, as will the amounts of each. To make this easier to think about, in the performance plate, we've split carbs into two groups: "Color," which refers to your fruits and vegetables, the brightly colored high fiber, high micronutrient options, and

"Carbs," which refers to things like bread, pasta and rice—think grains. It's important to note that especially on moderate to hard days, the carbs from your color aren't enough, and even on the low intensity and rest days, your plate should have some carbs!

LOW INTENSITY TRAINING AND REST DAYS

- Training Includes: Rest days, light body weight training, casual walks or jogs—this should all feel very easy
- Plate Should Be: Half colorful vegetables and fruits, a quarter carbohydrates, and a quarter protein plus fat

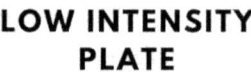
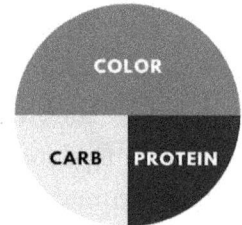

MODERATE INTENSITY TRAINING

- Training Includes: Most practices, most workouts, 1 hour or more strength training, 3+ mile runs—you're tired but not exhausted
- Plate Should Be: One-third vegetables and fruits, one-third carbohydrates, and one-third protein plus fat

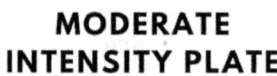
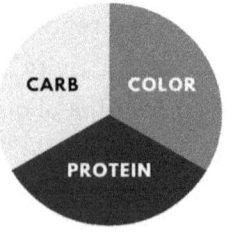

HIGH INTENSITY TRAINING

- Training Includes: Games or competition, tournaments, two-a-day practices, any workout above what's described in moderate training, or even any day where training just feels hard—you're tired and need to rest
- Plate Should Be: A quarter colorful vegetables and fruits, half carbohydrates, and a quarter protein plus fat

HIGH INTENSITY PLATE

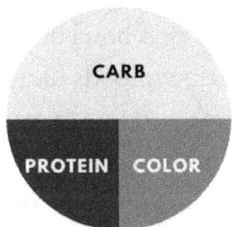

You'll notice that on the performance plates, we haven't included fat in the image. That's because it's rare that fat is on its own as a separate food. Instead, it's usually mixed in, either as the oil you use to sauté your vegetables or as part of your protein, since most animal-based protein sources contain fat. You *do* want to include fats at every meal, and you should be on the lookout to make sure that they're included, especially if you've been a low-fat athlete in the past or primarily eat plant-based, since you may need to shift your mindset around fat.

Again, for a day with light or no training, carbs are at their lowest, with one handful of carbohydrate, or about 25 percent of the plate. For moderate intensity activity, you'll see a plate that has about one and a half cupped hands of carbohydrate—closer to a third of the plate. For harder intensity days, it shifts to being two handfuls of carbs, taking up half of your plate. As the carbs shift, the amount of color and protein shift accordingly as well, in order to accommodate for those much-needed carbs.

If you're consistent with getting the right amount of nutrients you need in order for your body to perform at your best, you'll be amazed at the positive impact it can have on your performance, and on even on your body composition, since eating enough helps you ensure that you're building lean muscle.

We know this performance plate concept isn't always easy to use or follow. While this plate approach is great for a dinner like steak, rice and broccoli, it's not always so simple. What if it's not obvious how your meal breaks down onto a plate? It's much trickier to gauge how a meal stacks up in this breakdown if you're eating a sandwich, a piece of pizza or a bowl of stew or pasta. In those cases, you'll have to try to break down foods like this into their respective parts as best you can. It doesn't need to be perfect! For a couple slices of pizza, you're likely going to have one serving of carbs (a quarter of a plate) in each slice. Depending on your toppings, you may have vegetables to add to your color count, plus meat toppings that can count along with the cheese towards your protein count and fat count. Obviously, with something like pizza, your plate is going to be somewhat lacking in color—use that as a reminder to consider adding a side salad or some raw veggies, especially if you're eating a low intensity plate that day.

No matter what type of day you're fueling for, keep this in mind: Just say no to sad salads! You know the ones, the iceberg lettuce and balsamic vinegar as the entire meal. Salads should be tasty, nutrient-dense, and *actually* filling.

And remember: we don't need to micromanage our meals! The point of this exercise is to get better at gauging if you're eating *enough* at meals, not to test if you're doing everything perfectly. Your energy needs will swing from day to day, so rather than thinking about counting calories or even macros constantly, simply focus on building the appropriate plates for the work that you're doing.

WHAT YOU NEED TO KNOW ABOUT "ULTRA-PROCESSED," "PROCESSED" AND "UNPROCESSED" FOODS

When talking about what's on your plate, lately, the conversation has become less about the macronutrient breakdown and more about whether you have unprocessed or ultra-processed foods on the plate. You may have heard the terms unprocessed/whole, processed and ultra-processed in conversations about what's healthy and what isn't[i]. Often this breakdown gets explained as unprocessed being the healthiest and ultra-processed being very, very bad. For athletes in particular, it's a little more complicated.

While we love whole, unprocessed foods—again, bring on the big salad with a huge variety of veggies, nuts, seeds, chicken, olive oil and spices—athletes also need processed and ultra-processed carbohydrates to fuel training.

If you read or consume a lot of diet culture content, you likely associate things like cookies, cakes, bread, and bagels with being unhealthy, while you consider vegetables to be healthy. Fruit may fall somewhere in the middle. For athletes who need to fuel their training, it can be really difficult (arguably impossible) to do so eating only unprocessed, whole foods[ii]. To do that, your entire day essentially needs to be devoted to eating and training—and even then, you're still going to be adding in processed foods, since even raisins (dried fruit) and olive oil (pressed olives) count as 'processed.'

A few carbohydrate-rich processed and ultra-processed food sources for athletes include bagels, cereal, bread, pasta, rice, fruit, juice, and sports drinks, bars and gels. Notice a wide range of 'healthy' versus 'unhealthy' (or 'processed' versus 'ultra-processed') foods in there? Here's the thing: Especially when you're an athlete, but even simply as a young woman who's still developing and growing, you need a blend of foods. And almost none of them are inherently 'good' or 'bad.' Context—meaning how you're eating them and when you're eating them—matters. Plus, it's never a good idea to demonize one type of food by labeling it 'bad.'

It's also just plain confusing if you try to view food through this lens as an athlete. For example, maple syrup is a great example of a food that's all natural but would be considered processed because it's not in its natural form (tree sap), while a sports gel or bar would be considered ultra-processed since it's been formulated for maximum palatability. Both are great fuel for training. Some athletes love using maple syrup like a gel, for others, it hurts their stomach and they need a more specifically formulated sports drink. Either way, athletes need that fast fuel!

So rather than thinking about what you *don't* want, the goal should be to make sure you're getting a variety of foods for a variety of reasons. For example, when we think about some of our complex carbs like whole grains and vegetables, they provide fiber that can benefit heart health, regular bowel movements. We have high demands for that as an athlete. And then simple carbohydrates, like white bread and sports drinks, are going to be more easy to digest and better to time around our workouts. A blend of easy-to-digest carbohydrates like those in addition to the nutrient dense, fiber-rich carbs are both important for overall health. So stop adding value-based labels ("healthy" versus "unhealthy") to your foods and instead try to break them down to their macro and micronutrient content.

SPORT SPECIFICS

IN THIS SECTION, *it's time to develop smart eating strategies and habits to fuel the work you're doing at practice, whether you play a team sport, race for short distances, or tackle big endurance events. No matter what type of training or competition you're doing, fueling and hydrating right is the key to success.*

7 / PRE-WORKOUT FUELING

What should I eat before practice? What about before a big game? If I have a 5AM swim team session, do I need to wake up two hours early to eat breakfast? What foods should I avoid before training? Should I drink caffeine pre-game?

Eating ahead of training or competition is arguably the trickiest piece of the nutrition puzzle. Eat too much or eat the wrong thing for you and you risk heading to practice or onto the field feeling uncomfortably full with a rumbling gut that can send you rushing for the restrooms. Eat too little, and you're heading for a bonk, that lightheaded, low energy feeling that comes when your body is out of fuel. Neither of those situations is good. We're looking for a Goldilocks situation: The amount that's *just right*. Fortunately, with a bit of trial and error and determination, you *can* crack your fueling code.

Remember, what works for one person may not work for someone else, so don't assume your friend or teammate's fueling strategy is the winning one for you! Instead, try different options in practice, taking notes after each session about how your gut feels, and see what works best for you.

That said, there are some basic principles to get you started:

FUELING BEFORE PRACTICE

First and foremost, you have to fuel in order to train effectively. No matter what time of year it is, if training goes up, eating goes up. This means you can't afford to skip meals ahead of practices. Yes, that means even if you need to be on the pool deck at 5AM, you're going to need to sip on some sports drink or fruit juice, or have an easy-to-digest snack before you slip into the water.

We definitely want to be thinking about having some easy-to-digest carbohydrates before a workout, no matter what the workout is. We're not skipping meals. Even if it feels hard to eat and you're not hungry, you should be eating or drinking something before your workouts.

How much and what you eat is going to depend, since we all tolerate something different. What's going to work for you isn't going to work for somebody else: You may love oatmeal but it may make your teammate instantly need to poop!

Start to find what's right for you by testing out easy-to-digest carbohydrates like a banana, toast with jam, oatmeal with fruit, a bagel with peanut butter and honey, fig bars, applesauce pouches, or a sports drink. You may find that sipping a fruit juice (without pulp) is easy in the morning. If it sounds like something you like to eat or drink when your stomach hurts, it's likely a good pre-workout option! Trying different pre-workout snacks and meals is really important, because we're all going to tolerate something different. Spend a few weeks in the early season testing the different options and taking notes after practice about how you felt—start during low-key practices so that you're not scrambling when it's time for the big game. You'll start to figure out what's right for you.

No matter how solid your gut is, two hours ahead of a workout, you really want to limit fat, fiber and protein in your food, because those things will slow down digestion and can lead to having an upset stomach during your practice[i].

Your first sip of water shouldn't come 10 minutes into practice when your coach calls for a break! In addition to fueling, we also want to hydrate ahead of practice—not so much that you're peeing every five minutes, but enough that you're not starting mildly dehydrated. Just sip from a water bottle as you make your way to practice. (This is easy if you're using a sports drink to fuel, since it does double duty.)

If your practice is later in the day or after dinner, you'll want to eat normally at meal times throughout the day, prioritizing carbs but also getting plenty of protein, fat and fiber. Then, in the two to three hours before practice, dial down the fat and fiber and focus on carbs that feel good in your gut. This can be tricky to get used to if you're typically someone who does cereal for breakfast, a salad for lunch, and a big dinner with lots of meat and veggies. You may have to start shifting those meals so that breakfast is a veggie-filled omelette with potatoes and toast, lunch is a wrap with veggies and protein, and pre-workout dinner is actually more like your 'standard' breakfast, with toast or cereal. (If you're eating most meals in the dining hall, consider sneaking in a plastic container to fill with your dinner cereal or peanut butter and jelly bagel. We won't tell!)

How much should you eat? It's going to depend on what your workout or competition looks like[ii]. Here's how you can think about your pre-workout snack[iii], depending on what training you have on tap:

- For a 15-45 min workout: 15-30 grams of carbs – a snack like a banana or a handful of cereal will do the trick
- For a 30-60 min workout: 30-60 grams of carbs – e.g., toast with jam or a fruit smoothie
- For a 60+ min workout: 60-90 grams of carbs – e.g., oatmeal with fruit or a bagel with peanut butter + honey
- For a 90+ min workout: ≥ 90 grams of carbs. In this case, you should also be increasing your carb intake the day before (an extra serving of pasta, bread and rice at dinner

are some ideas), then topping up with a carb-rich pre-run meal

Fueling for practice doesn't start with the meal or snack right before training, it should be considered an all-day, all-the-time thing, especially if you're an athlete who's putting in 10+ hours of training each week. We often say that if you're waiting until the night before the race to start carb-loading, you've waited too long to dial in your nutrition. *Every* meal is an opportunity to boost your recovery and to start prepping for the next practice.

FUELING BEFORE A COMPETITION

Getting ready for a big game or an everyday training session should actually look very similar. Think of your training sessions as a chance not just to practice the skills and speed you need for competition, but a chance to practice the fueling aspect as well. That way, on race or game day, there are no surprises.

The only difference between your normal pre-workout meal and a competition day one is that you want to stick to what you know even more closely during a competition—and this can be complicated if you're traveling to compete. Because of that, if you know most games/races are 'away,' get your gut used to foods that are easy to access anywhere. Toast, cereal, instant oats, bagels, bananas—these are all easy to access at most hotel breakfast buffets or supermarkets. It is also good to have a simple bar or another pre-packaged easy to grab and pack carb source like applesauce packets, fig bars or granola bars that you've used in practice and can work in a pinch. That way, you'll have a backup that you can always have on hand.

YOUR PRE-COMPETITION FUELING TIMELINE

- 3-4 Hours: Have a meal using the High Intensity Performance Plate (half of the plate should be carbs, make sure it's low in fat).
- 2 Hours: Have a balanced snack that pairs one to two servings of carbs with a serving of protein, avoiding fat and fiber.
- 60-90 Minutes: Choose a carb-rich snack that's one to two servings of easy to digest carb (can be in drink form). Avoid fat, fiber and protein.
- 45 Minutes or Less: Get some fast fuel. This is fast-digesting carb-based sports drinks, fruit juice or other simple carbohydrate source. Must be low in fat, fiber and protein.

THE TRUTH ABOUT ENERGY SUPPLEMENTS

Outside of a cup of coffee at breakfast, I don't recommend pre-workout "energy" supplements or powders[iv] for a few reasons. These products often contain high levels of caffeine, which can lead to unwanted side effects, like anxiety, tremors, heart palpitations, chest pains, seizures, and even death. Many of them aren't third-party tested, which means you're also at risk of ingesting banned substances. And some products have certain ingredients like beetroot that can actually cause digestive upset in some athletes.

For adults over 18, 400 milligrams of caffeine per day is the maximum amount recommended. If you're between 13 and 18, the American Academy of Pediatrics recommends under 100 milligrams of caffeine per day—about a cup of coffee. If you're under 12, definitely skip caffeine altogether!

Assuming you're over 12, caffeine itself isn't entirely bad or something that must be avoided, but you do need to be cautious about the amount and the timing of the caffeine that you're consuming. A single cup of coffee may make you feel more alert and act as a performance enhancer, but two cups may make you jittery and actually decrease your performance. Many energy drinks contain several cups of coffee's worth of caffeine, which is why we don't recommend them.

Everyone metabolizes caffeine differently[v]: If you're someone who's a slow metabolizer, it can take hours for the effects of an espresso shot or energy drink to wear off, so especially if you have late in the day practices, proceed with caution where caffeine is concerned. If you struggle with sleep issues, definitely check in on your caffeine intake and timing.

Pay attention to how that coffee makes you feel immediately after drinking it, but also a couple of hours later. Finally, it's worth noting that too much caffeine can also lead to a positive drug test if you're in a collegiate sport that uses NCAA standards for anti-doping[vi].

I get it: Many of us—myself included—rely on that morning cup of coffee. However, if on a daily basis, you can't do anything without that coffee, that's a big red flag that something needs to change in your schedule or your meal planning, since caffeine reliance is a sign that you need more rest and recovery along with more energy from actual food. It's easy to forget that food provides the body energy, as does proper rest. So, if you're regularly feeling your energy crash and slump in the afternoon, try reaching for a snack or taking a short nap before grabbing that energy drink or afternoon coffee.

EXAMPLES OF EASY PRE-WORKOUT SNACKS

Pre-workout, in addition to water and coffee (in moderation), we recommend drinking a generic sports drink if you're going to have anything sport-specific. Gatorade is the obvious option that's available pretty much anywhere, but you can also cut fruit juice with water and add a pinch of salt for bonus sodium. These are great options to help hydrate while providing a bit of energy:

- Fig Bars (2-4)

- Fresh Fruit (2 whole pieces or 2 cups)
- Dried Fruit (1/3 to 1/2 cup)
- 100% Fruit Juice (1 cup)
- White bagel (1/2 to 1 bagel or 1-2 mini bagels)
- White bread (2 slices)
- Nonfat/low-fat yogurt with fruit (1 cup yogurt + 1 cup fruit)
- English Muffin (1-2 muffins)
- Applesauce Packets (1-2 packets)
- Cereal with Milk (1 cup cereal + 3/4 cup nonfat or low-fat milk)
- Homemade Fruit Smoothie (1-2 cups fruit, 1 cup nonfat or low-fat milk or yogurt)
- Frozen Waffles (2 or 1 with fruit/syrup topping)
- Pretzels (handful)
- White rice (1 cup)
- Potato (1 medium)
- Energy Waffles (Honey Stinger, 2 waffles)
- Sports Chews (Clif Bloks, Gatorade Prime, Honey Stinger Chews)
- Sports Drinks (Gatorade, Powerade - full sugar, 2-3 cups)
- Sports Gel (1-2 packets)

8 / DURING TRAINING + COMPETITION

DURING A WORKOUT, a race or a competition, there are two primary objectives when it comes to fueling: Drink enough water and take in enough electrolytes to maintain a healthy hydration status *and* take in enough simple carbohydrates to fuel the work that you're doing. Fueling during a workout also helps us recover faster.

However, depending on the practice, training or competition, the way that you fuel and how much you take in will vary dramatically from sport to sport. The way you fuel a long run—a steady state of constant movement over the course of hours—will look much different from the way you would fuel a track workout that's defined by short, fast efforts with breaks in between, or from the way you would fuel a soccer practice where you're running up and down the field in inconsistent bursts of energy, even though in all three cases, you're running *a lot*. Here, we're breaking it down as simply as we can, but if it seems confusing, remember this key piece of information:

When in doubt, sip some water and eat a bite of something, or take a sip of a sports drink. It's always better to fuel more rather than less.

FUELING WITH CARBS

For athletes, sugar is an excellent fuel source for you. But if you skipped reading the 'Carbs Are Queen' chapter, you may still be under the mistaken impression that sugar is bad, *period*. You may have been told (likely by some bro who considers himself a 'nutrition expert who does his own research') that sports drinks, gels and bars are bad for you, or seen one of your parents attempt a low carb or no carb diet. But athletes are unique compared to the average or sedentary person who is not exercising or training regularly for extended periods of time. Simple sugars, specifically glucose and fructose, are very efficient fuel sources during exercise[i].

Your body has a certain amount of energy stored, but it still needs help, especially as intensity or duration of exercise increases. By consuming simple sugars during exercise, you're not depleting your body of its stored form of carbohydrate—glycogen[ii]—all the time. The more we rely on that stored form of carbohydrate, the more depleted we get. Yes, you'll be able to keep going for a while, but eventually, you'll start to fade. Even if you're taking in carbs, you'll still be dipping into those glycogen stores, because it's really hard to fuel fast enough to replace all of them. That supply is not endless, and the more we rely on it heavily, it will also impact not just our performance, but also our ability to recover.

Your body needs to restock its glycogen stores you've used up: If you're constantly running on empty during training and then not eating enough during the rest of the day, your body just can't get ahead. And often, in those cases we start to see a lot of soreness, poor recovery after workouts, interrupted sleep, mood disturbances, and irritability. The best way to help your body refill those glycogen stores is to avoid depleting them as much as possible.

Have you tried fueling in the past and been plagued with stomach issues? Part of the reason why you might have these stomach issues with fueling during exercise is because physiologically, when you're exercising, your body is not prioritizing digestion, so it's struggling to break down your food. Your body is prioritizing getting oxygen and nutrients to your working muscles so you can keep moving. Because of that, it slows down digestion. That's why what you eat or drink matters. Fat, fiber, and protein slow down digestion, which makes them not ideal for consuming during exercise. Having easy-to-digest carbohydrates[iii] rather than more 'whole food' type options is important during exercise. Simple sugars like those found in fruit juice, maple syrup, honey, white rice and simple carbohydrate-based sports fuels and products are really great tools for us, because they are designed for your body to break them down very easily and be used for energy right away. The other reason you may have dealt with gut distress is because your body simply isn't used to being fed during exercise. For some people, this does need to be trained, the same way you need to put in reps in the gym to get stronger.

HYDRATION 101

When it comes to hydration, we're not just talking about drinking enough water, we're also talking about the important role electrolytes play in being properly hydrated. The combination of water and electrolytes, especially sodium—either mixed into your water or eaten in your food—is what creates optimal fluid balance in your body. And as with most things in nutrition, it's pretty darn individual, but there are some basic principles.

We don't need to tell you that you need water in order to survive. During exercise, you lose water primarily due to sweat but also through aspiration (breathing), and it needs to be replaced.

Electrolytes are a bit more complex. They're minerals that have a natural positive or negative electrical charge when dissolved in water, and include sodium, potassium, chloride, magnesium, calcium, phosphate, and bicarbonates. These help your body regulate different chemical reactions and maintain the balance between fluids in and outside of your cells.

We lose electrolytes when we sweat—that's why sweat tastes salty, and why some saltier sweaters end up with white marks on clothing or gritty feeling skin, especially on hot and humid days. It is important that we maintain electrolyte balance, and that means we need to take in electrolytes to replace the ones we sweat out.

The amount of electrolytes you need will vary from athlete to athlete, and it's weather and temperature dependent as well as effort-level dependent. In our sweat, we primarily lose sodium, chloride, potassium and calcium. Everybody is going to have a different base-line sweat composition: Some people may lose more electrolytes in their sweat. It's genetic[iv]. Sodium is going to be the electrolyte we lose most generously in sweat, which is why you'll hear about it in the context of replacing it as an athlete. The other three aren't as important to replace instantly, since you lose them in smaller quantities and they don't impact performance as dramatically. But if you're sweating out too much sodium, you'll start to notice a performance decline.

The next question to ask is: How do you know if you are a salty sweater? Sweat composition is genetic, so it's fairly consistent, even if your sweat rate changes based on external factors like temperature. Some people are saltier sweaters, some people are not. You can sweat large amounts and not be a salty sweater. Some people lose a lot of water during exercise but only a small amount of sodium. But others lose sodium at a rapid rate, which can decrease performance and make you more susceptible to hyponatremia. There are signs that you might be a salty sweater and need to really focus on your electrolyte intake during training[v]: You may notice frequent stomach pain like cramping, decreased performance as you sweat (unless you're replacing fluids and electrolytes well), and even having lower tolerance to the heat can be a sign. You may notice grittiness or salt rings on your gear after hot practices. In that case, what's happening is your sweat is evaporating and leaving that salt behind.

We talk about water and electrolytes together because they impact each other so much. Electrolytes play a big role in making sure our body is properly hydrated. Dehydration and low electrolyte levels aren't the same thing but they are related, because electrolytes are key to maintaining fluid balance and making sure we're properly hydrated. If you drink a lot of water but don't take in enough electrolytes, your body can't actually use that water effectively, so even though you're drinking 'enough,' your hydration status may be suffering. In fact, too much water with too low electrolyte levels can be fatal—you may have heard of deaths in marathons from hyponatremia, which is when the concentration of sodium in your blood is abnormally low, often because an athlete is fueling with just water, and too much of it. Symptoms of hyponatremia[vi] include confusion, fatigue, headache, irritability, muscle weakness, spasms, and cramps. When it's becoming more acute, it can shift to nausea, vomiting, and seizures, potentially ending in death.

Don't be scared of hydrating, though! We need to account for what fluids we're losing when we sweat, so we need appropriate amounts of water. Dehydration is also dangerous—and can cause serious declines in your performance[vii].

How can you tell if you're not hydrating enough? You might finish your run or ride and feel drained the rest of the day, or experience muscle cramps during or after exercise. You might get nausea or have that 'splashy stomach' feeling.

You can also use a scale to get a better sense of how much fluid you're losing during activity so you know how much to drink. Hop on a scale before you train, pay attention to how much water you take in during training, and weigh yourself after.

Total Sweat Loss = pre-weight - post-weight + weight of water consumed
[Your weight pre-exercise] - [Your weight post-exercise] + [The weight of fluid consumed (convert ounces to pounds by dividing the ounces by 16)] = Total sweat lost during exercise
Example: 130 pounds at start of soccer practice - 128 pounds after practice + 2 pounds (32 ounces of water) = 4 pounds (64 ounces) of water lost during practice

In sport, we're aiming to replace 50 to 75 percent of the fluid you lose per hour, plus around 300 to 600 milligrams of sodium[viii,ix,x]. So in that example above, ideally we'd be drinking 16 to 24 ounces of water per hour plus 300 to 600 milligrams of sodium per hour during that session.

Your university may offer sweat rate testing for athletes, and if it does, definitely take advantage of that option! It can be very beneficial for an endurance athlete in particular to look at their sweat rate, especially if you tend to have post-run headaches, issues like bloating and GI distress during and after training, or you feel like your performance really declines in heat.

One final note: Don't let this section convince you that you need electrolytes in your water all day, every day. Drinking regular water during the day and saving electrolytes for before and during training is ideal for most people. If you love a particular electrolyte tablet or powder, it's not going to hurt, but it's likely not necessary outside of training. Just make sure that most of your regular meals include a sprinkle of salt, especially if you steer clear of processed foods and sauces, which typically contain more sodium.

FUELING TEAM/INDOOR SPORTS

These guidelines are for sports with frequent breaks in practice or competition where you'll be able to access a bottle and any snacks you need. This includes softball, soccer, gymnastics, track and field, rugby, and even swimming. It can also apply to the weight room.

- **Goal**: Stay hydrated and snack when necessary
- **Target**: 16 to 20-ounce bottle of water/sports drink per hour (include electrolytes in the form of sports drink that includes sodium and potassium or by adding a pinch of salt to water) and fuel with 30-60 grams of carbohydrates per hour[xi]

- **Easy options for fuel:** Bananas, pretzels, cookies, crackers, cereal, sports drink mix, water mixed with apple or grape juice in a 2:1 ratio

During the practice or game, use any pauses in activity to take a bite and a drink. (Or just a drink, if you use a sports drink for your carbohydrates and electrolytes as well as hydration.)

Pay attention to signs of dehydration, which can include struggling to focus, headache, gut distress or even just feeling 'off.' If you start feeling 'not great,' think about the last time you had some water, electrolytes and carbs. If it's been a while, it's time to take a drink. And yes, you can get dehydrated even in the pool!

You shouldn't end a practice or competition feeling like you need to eat or drink immediately or you'll fall over. Yes, you may be hungry, but you shouldn't be ravenous. If you are, that's a sign that you need to eat more during your event.

FUELING ENDURANCE SPORTS

These guidelines are for sports that don't typically include pauses in activity and require a sustained effort. This includes running, biking, hiking, and swimming.

- **Goal**: Stay hydrated and snack when necessary
- **Target**: 20-ounce bottle of water per hour, 60-90 grams of carbohydrates per hour[xii], include electrolytes in the form of sports drink that includes sodium and potassium or by adding a pinch of salt to water
- **Easy options for fuel:** Bananas, cookies, homemade rice bars, sport-specific gels, bars and drink mixes (these differ from team sport options because they need to be a bit easier to eat since you're eating while in motion)

The transition from team sports to endurance training is tricky. If you're used to being a track athlete who focuses on the 200-meter and suddenly you're going for the 10,000-meter, you'll need to change your fueling approach for those long runs. It can be tough, going from sipping water on the sideline to suddenly needing to think about bringing a handheld bottle for your hour-long run.

Even for shorter endurance training sessions—under an hour—you should still think about fueling. You technically can get away with an easy hour-long ride or run without fuel or hydration (unless it's super hot out, in which case you do actually need that bottle!), but it's better to get in the fueling habit and be well-fueled rather than chronically underfueled, which unfortunately, is where most young women fall on the fueling-during-sport spectrum.

When you get home from a run or a bike ride, your goal is to feel like you could eat… but not that you have to immediately. You should be able to comfortably take a shower and clean up, then make yourself a recovery meal. If you feel the urge to shove your head into a bag of chips or bowl of ice cream, that's a good sign that you didn't fuel enough.

You can get better at fueling in two main ways: First, fuel every training session, even the easy ones. This gets your gut and brain used to the fuel you're using and to the idea of regularly fueling. It also lets you start to work out how much fuel makes you feel your best. You can practice what fuel you want to use, trying different flavors, different textures and different products, and in doing so, you're also training your gut to tolerate more fuel, because almost no one is going to wake up and tolerate 60 to 90 grams of carbs per hour during exercise without any practice. Most people need to work up to that, so these shorter runs or rides or workouts can be a good opportunity to practice getting a little bit more and starting to train your gut to tolerate that fuel source.

Second, take good notes! Wherever you keep your notes about your training, whether it's a written training log, spreadsheet, Strava, Training Peaks or some other software, write down what you ate and drank and how you felt. This helps you start to spot patterns and hone in on the foods that work best for your gut, and how much fuel you need for your best energy levels.

WHAT TO AVOID DURING WORKOUTS

There are a few things to avoid eating or drinking during workouts that can lead to serious tummy trouble, and unless you love doing the port-a-potty sprint, check the ingredients on your snacks before practice!

During a workout, I recommend avoiding anything with any artificial sweeteners. They aren't helpful, and unfortunately, they're often replacing sugar, which we need for energy. But second, artificial sweeteners can also cause some gut upset. (For more on artificial sweeteners, check out the Carbs Are Queen chapter).

We also want to try and avoid fiber in the context of a workout. It's great at all other times, but fiber slows down digestion, and that's going to lead to gut issues if you're trying to train with a lot of fiber in your tummy. This sounds strange—who's crunching on kale during a workout?—but a lot of people equate packets of baby food or pureed dates with sports gels. And both of those things are incredibly high in fiber. Fig bars are another potentially tricky snack: A small amount might be fine, but too many can be too much fiber. The same is true of fruit juice that contains pulp.

Too much fat and protein can also be a problem for digestion, because again, they take longer to digest and also don't provide fast, accessible fuel for your muscles. A little bit of fat or protein in a bar is fine, but a protein bar or shake during a workout will do more harm than good.

FUELING SPORT ON A TIGHT BUDGET

Dining halls are the perfect spot to snag free workout fuel. We won't tell anyone! Bring your water bottle and a few plastic baggies to breakfast and stock up. A few of our favorites:

- Sweetened iced tea
- Fruit juice mixed in a 2:1 ratio with water
- Sports drink (yes, some dining halls have Gatorade at the soda fountain!)
- Graham crackers
- Peanut butter + jelly sandwiches
- Bagels
- Toast with jam
- Packets of jam
- Maple syrup or honey (bonus points if you BYO plastic flask to fill!)
- Cereal
- White rice
- Bananas
- Oranges
- Cookies

9 / POST-WORKOUT FUELING

AFTER YOUR PRACTICE, workout, gym session or competition, it's time to focus on recovery, which we'll refer to as post-workout for the rest of the chapter. Post-workout, your body needs carbohydrates to replace the stores that it burned up during training, and it needs protein to kickstart muscle repair and growth. It also needs water to replace any lost during the workout.

Yes, the myth that you only have 30 minutes post-workout to eat or you'll miss out on all the gains has been debunked. But while it may not be biologically true, it's still a good idea from a practical standpoint.

After your workout, aim for around a 3-to-1 ratio of carbohydrates to protein[i]. That looks like 60 grams of carbohydrate (about 240 calories) with 20 grams of protein (about 80 calories) as your starting point. That amount of carbs and protein should increase if you had a harder or longer workout, but begin there. And again, make sure you're drinking some water along with your snack.

If that feels complicated, go even simpler. What are things that you like that you can very easily grab post-workout? Is it chocolate milk and a banana? Is it a yogurt-based smoothie that you can make quickly? What about a bowl with Greek yogurt or cottage cheese with berries, granola, and honey? Find a combination of the carbs and protein that works for you, and you'll be replenishing that muscle glycogen, the stored form of carbohydrate, as well as kickstarting muscle repair and recovery. Once you have a post-training formula figured out, stick to it—boring is good, in this case!

A lot of athletes opt for liquid recovery in the form of drink mixes, smoothies, shakes or even our favorite, chocolate milk. That's not because liquid is better for your recovery, it's just that it's often easier and faster for an athlete to grab-and-go, and it allows you to refuel and rehydrate at the same time. In fact, we tend to not love recovery powders and mixes because they're quite expensive for what they are. They work fine, but chocolate milk or a smoothie with yogurt would work just as well. But the recovery drink mixes are nice to have if you're in a pinch and just don't have time to make something else. Think of them as just one tool in your toolbox.

Some people who struggle with their appetites or feel nauseous or not hungry after their training sessions can benefit from those liquid choices. It can be very hard to eat and consume things when you feel that way, but we still need to get that nutrition on board and start the recovery process.

If you prefer a solid meal and have time to have one, that's great. It's just about preference and what you'll actually do on a regular basis.

Speaking of solid meals, should you count post workout recovery as a meal if you're eating it at your usual breakfast, lunch or dinner time? Or should it be a bonus meal? It's absolutely fine to just eat lunch as usual if your workout ends at 11:30AM—but if that's the case, consider adding in a snack between lunch and dinner to top off those energy stores.

This is a common issue for athletes who are struggling with low energy availability: Using a regular meal as a recovery meal means missing the chance to add extra carbohydrates and protein to your daily intake, and that can put you into a chronic low energy state. In fact, a lot of athletes who are somewhat stealthily trying to limit calories may try to time workouts so that they coincide with mealtimes in order to avoid needing that extra snack. But that will backfire on you eventually. (We'll talk more about that later.)

If your next meal is an hour after your workout, don't wait. Use that immediate post-workout time to have something small as well. It doesn't have to be much! Again, think simple: a yogurt, chocolate milk, or a handful of pretzels or a banana with peanut butter.

On double workout days in particular, three meals just isn't going to be enough. You're going to need to get some snacks in there. Bring a smoothie or even just a chocolate milk with you to class if you're pressed for time and can't sit down to an extra meal.

Personally, I like to view snacks as opportunities! They're a great way to help meet your higher energy and micronutrient needs without the overwhelm or stress of sitting down to huge meals. It can be hard to eat a lot of volume in one sitting, so those snacks help meet those higher energy demands. Snacks also keep you more energized throughout the day.

A few signs you need to snack more:

- If you start to feel tired or lose focus or attention in class in the afternoon, that is a very good indicator that you didn't eat enough earlier in the day. Try adding in a mid-morning snack and see how you feel.
- If you're waking up really hungry in the morning or even at night, it's time to add a bonus bedtime snack.
- If you're having trouble sleeping (getting to sleep or staying asleep), adding in that bedtime snack is often the answer.

Remember: As training goes up, eating goes up. And that means both in practice and out of practice. In fact, typically as training volume or intensity goes up, you won't necessarily be able to consume significantly more during your training, so most of the fuel increases should take place before and after workouts.

The biggest mistake I see young athletes make is skipping the post-workout immediate refuel because they're rushing to get to the next class or work. If you've fallen out of that good habit of doing a post-workout immediate refuel, that's an easy piece of the puzzle to put back in place. Skipping that refuel often starts innocently—you're having lunch in 90 minutes, so you'll just wait. But life gets in the way, and suddenly, lunch gets skipped and now it's been four hours since you trained and you still haven't refueled. And that's a problem.

A FEW SIMPLE RECOVERY SNACK FAVORITES

- Chocolate Milk (1.5-2 cups)
- Bagel + Peanut Butter, Cream Cheese, or String Cheese
- Cottage Cheese + Fruit
- Greek Yogurt + Fruit and/or Honey
- Peanut Butter + Jelly/Honey Sandwich
- Turkey Sandwich
- Hummus and Pretzels
- Protein bar (at least 10 gram protein) + Fruit
- Dried Fruit + String Cheese
- Pasta + Chicken
- Avocado Toast + Fruit
- Fig Bars or Rice Cakes + Protein Shake
- Whole Grain Crackers + Peanut/Almond Butter
- Nuts + Fruit
- Grilled Cheese Sandwich + Fruit
- Ready-To-Drink Recovery Beverages

Don't forget to add a bottle of water, fruit juice or sports drink!

WHAT ABOUT THE OFFSEASON?

A lot of athletes see the offseason as a chance to lose weight and to decrease their intake. But don't think that the offseason is the time to throw this book away! You need to fuel properly in the offseason as well. There may be slight adjustments to how you're eating if your training load has significantly decreased, but these should be small changes, not major restrictions.

As athletes, we still need to eat a solid amount overall. We just might not need that extra snack or two. In the offseason, we're definitely not avoiding entire food groups. We are absolutely not restricting carbohydrates. We are not neglecting fueling before, during and after our strength and conditioning sessions. If we're still going to the pool or the track, even if those training sessions in the offseason are lighter, we're still eating before them, fueling during them, and refueling after.

I see a lot of athletes do this wrong. Their training cuts back and they automatically think, 'Oh, I'm not training as much. I don't need to eat before this 40 minute lift because it's not a two hour practice like I'm used to.' But you still need to fuel those shorter efforts appropriately and make sure that you're not cutting corners in the name of weight loss.

Your approach should always be that during the offseason, you're supporting your body so it can recover from the past season and all the work you did during it. You're also continuing to support your body through the lower training volume, because you're still going to school, still doing all of your other extracurricular activities, still growing, still using your glycogen-burning brain, still dealing with all of those other demands that you're putting on your body... and remember, you also need to come into next season feeling your best. Restricting won't get you there.

10 / COMMON DIGESTIVE ISSUES

I CAN'T EAT before practice, it makes me feel nauseous! How do I prevent stomach issues during competition? I'm having burping, heartburn and a tight chest when I run at rugby practice after I have a meal—should I take something? Can you be hungover from eating pizza? Should I need to hit the bathroom every five minutes when I'm running?

Digestion should be a simple process: Put food and water in, use what you need, eventually poop out what you don't need. But sadly, it's often not that simple for athletes, especially young women who are juggling sport, school, work and life, often eating at less-than-ideal times. Hormones also play a role in digestion[i], meaning sometimes during the month throughout your menstrual cycle, everything can be running smoothly... And then, other weeks, you're sprinting for the locker room bathroom part way through practice.

So, let's talk about digestion—the good, the bad and the, well, extremely uncomfortable.

Unfortunately, a lot of athletes—especially women—deal with a lot of gut distress on a regular basis[ii]. It's so regular, in fact, that they eventually just start to consider it 'normal.' But here's the deal: While some gut distress like stomach cramps or diarrhea or nausea *occasion-*

ally is nothing to worry about, if you're regularly experiencing bloating, cramping, diarrhea, constipation, nausea, gas, acid reflux, or any other kind of stomach distress, that shouldn't be considered normal. It should be taken as a sign that something is going on with your gut.

That said, don't freak out. This is actually good news! If you can crack your gut's code and understand what it's trying to tell you, you'll not only be able to work on the root causes of those symptoms, you'll also likely see an improvement in your athletic performance. The runner who isn't frantically searching out a port-a-potty mid-marathon and who is able to fuel herself adequately without fear of that feeling will almost certainly have a better finishing time.

But what is "Good Digestion," anyway? Start by contemplating your poop.

Yes, you read that right. Having optimized poop most of the time is generally a sign that things are going well in your gut. If your poop isn't ideal—if you're on the constipated side or you tend to have a lot of loose stool—that's a sign there's a chronic issue to address.

Consistency-wise, the Bristol Stool Chart[iii] is the gold standard for getting a read on your bowel movements. The ideal poop is a smooth sausage shape with minimal surface cracks. It shouldn't be liquid-y, nor should it be hard clumps.

Bristol Stool Chart

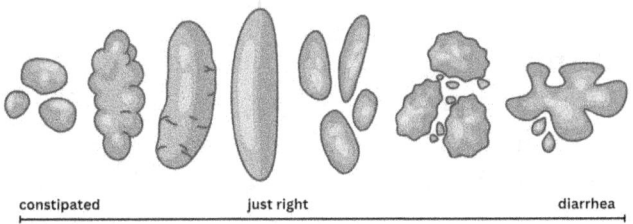

constipated · just right · diarrhea

Color-wise, we're looking for medium to dark brown poop. Black, white, green, red, orange, yellow stools all can be indicative of some other problem that might be happening—definitely check with a doctor if you notice anything like that! Well, check with a doctor *unless* you ate something out-of-the-ordinary and stool color is your only issue. Your food can sometimes cause funky colors in your poop. Eating a lot of beets or putting beet juice in your smoothie can make stool and urine go red, which is alarming to say the least! But if there's any pain or discomfort plus a funky color, even if you think it's from something you ate, err on the side of caution and check with a doctor.

Ease of pooping is also key for good gut health. You shouldn't be straining: It shouldn't be a huge effort to go. It definitely shouldn't hurt when you poop. And generally speaking, you should be pooping at least once every day[iv]. There are some situations where this isn't the case, but if you're an exception to that rule, you've likely already had this discussion with a doctor!

Not pooping regularly, or struggling when you do, and you're not sure why? For most young women, a lack of dietary fiber can be a huge player in irregular or not normal bowel movements. Athletes in particular are susceptible to this since it can be made worse by dehydration, even very mild dehydration. Your body requires enough liquid to move the stool through the digestive tract easily, and fiber gives it the bulk it needs to make its way out. But between losing water to our training when we sweat, which leads to dehydration, and skipping fiber-rich meals because we're trying to fuel our training with simple carbs, it's easy to end up on the wrong side of this equation.

Fiber is tricky for athletes. To recap from our carb chapter, there are two different types of fiber that are key for digestion, soluble and insoluble. Soluble fiber dissolves in water and forms a gel-like substance during digestion, slowing down the digestive process (which is a good thing since it gives the body time to process nutrients). Insoluble fiber does *not* dissolve in water and it adds bulk to the stool to help move food through the digestive system more quickly. We need both: soluble fiber helps with nutrient absorption, blood sugar control and cholesterol levels while insoluble fiber helps you poop better and move the extra 'stuff' out of your system.

If you're eating enough overall and balancing your performance plates well, the optimal fiber intake is pretty easy to hit. Make sure you're getting that color—those fruits and veggies—on most plates and you should be good to go, pun intended. However, beware of overdoing it on fiber, especially around training, since too much fiber in your gut typically leads to bloating and cramping during exercise. The same applies to if you're taking a fiber supplement rather than just eating fiber-rich foods. In fact, please don't try that—you can get plenty of fiber, along with other nutrients, from food!

The other major factor that leads to gut issues is ironically not eating *enough*. Not eating enough in general, especially over a longer period of time, is going to do some horrible things to your stomach[v]. Chronic underfueling can cause a lot of digestive issues during exercise and outside of exercise[vi,vii]. I find that a lot of athletes only experience gut distress during exercise, and because of that, they like to blame the sports drink or the gel or what they had before training. But often, underfueling overall is to blame. This is because over time, if you're chronically underfueled, your body doesn't have the energy and resources to meet the demands of exercise, training, recovery and growth, as well as the other things like mental demands of school and life. Forget about digestion! There are a lot of energy demands in your body, and when the energy demands are high but we're not meeting them with our fueling, we end up with gut issues because our body doesn't have the resources that it needs, and those issues become more noticeable during exercise.

When your body's not getting the energy and resources it needs, it is going to start to prioritize the most important things. Think of it like your body is going to start cutting corners. Digestion is an energy-demanding process[viii], so your body will slow that process down, and then if you add exercise on top of that, that exercise increases inflammation in the body, which will also create inflammation in your gut, which will then create digestive issues. Yikes.

It's also a vicious cycle: If it hurts after you eat or it hurts to train with anything in your stomach, guess what? You're unlikely to eat enough, because you're trying to avoid that pain. So, poor digestion can also exacerbate issues like REDs and LEA in athletes[ix]. (More on REDs and LEA in chapter 13.)

If you've decided to eliminate an entire food group from your diet to try to heal your gut without any testing or working with a dietitian, you may want to re-evaluate. I've seen a lot of athletes who eliminated gluten and dairy thinking they were *solving* their digestive issues, but they actually *added* to those issues, since the real problem was underfueling, and cutting out those food groups made the situation even worse!

For example, there are a lot of athletes who cut out gluten in recent years, and for some, that was a necessary, positive choice. But there were a lot of athletes who really didn't need to eliminate it, but who did because their friends or teammates were doing it, and many of them subsequently struggled with underfueling. Whenever an athlete eliminates a major food group, it automatically puts athletes at a higher risk for underfueling. Yes, sometimes there is a medical necessity, but in these cases, a doctor or dietitian should be involved. (If you're not sure about if you have a food intolerance, registered dietitians are able to use protocols like GI Mapping or supervised elimination diets that can help you better pinpoint your problem foods[x].)

So, if all of this sounds like you, it's time to start adding, not subtracting. When you have gut issues, the tendency is to eat less, but in reality, you need to be eating more! But focus on small steps, not huge changes. You don't have to go zero to 100, but where can you start to slowly increase intake? Maybe you aren't eating before practice: Can you sip a sports drink or eat half of a banana before practice? What about after practice: Can you add a recovery shake or chocolate milk? If you are not used to consuming *anything* during exercise, start really small. Even small amounts are going to impact your performance positively. So start small, try different flavors, try different textures.

If you do believe that you're eating enough in and out of training but still dealing with gut distress, yes, it could be the sports drink, gel or bar that you're consuming. Not every drink mix is going to work well for every athlete. So try something different!

Start by checking that whatever you're using is extremely low in anything other than carbohydrates: Make sure there's no fat, protein or fiber hiding in there! Those can slow down digestion and cause that distress. People can also be very sensitive to flavors, textures and levels of sweetness, so it can take some experimentation to find what works best for you.

And yes, there is too much of a good thing. If you're taking in too much during exercise, you may have issues like stomach cramps, nausea, bloating, diarrhea, and general discomfort. That's why I suggest starting small and slowly adding more when it comes to fueling, because you need to find where your body is happiest digestion-wise. When you're exercising, there's reduced blood flow to your gut, so the blood is going to be diverted to your working muscles and away from your gut. That means instead of focusing on digestion, your body is prioritizing running or kicking the ball. Because of this, the digestion process gets slowed down. Sports drinks, gels and bars are designed to be easy to digest, but if you're taking in too much, it can still back your system up.

We're big fans of sports drinks or fruit juice for new-to-consuming-calories athletes, since those are the easiest to digest and come with the hydration that you also need to speed up digestion and absorption. Simple candy like gummy bears can be great as well—and it's fun to eat!

Good digestion is also related to understanding our body's hunger cues, and honoring them by eating when we're hungry. But as athletes, leaning into hunger cues is a complicated topic since sometimes, we do need to override what our body seems like it's saying and just have the snack, sports drink, gel, whatever. Hunger cues simply do not count in and around training[xi]. But especially outside of our actual training, we want to learn to tune into our bodies.

Think of hunger and fullness on a scale of one to 10. We want to generally stay at between a four and a seven on the scale, so we're not letting ourselves get so hungry that we're cranky, but also not get uncomfortably full.

We want to learn our hunger cues and listen to our bodies, but using hunger cues instead of eating in a more scheduled way can be a sneaky way of getting restrictive with our eating. If you've been restricting calories for a long time, you may not have obvious hunger cues[xii]—why would your body scream if no one is going to listen? If you have a history of eating disorders or disordered eating, telling yourself that you're "just listening to hunger cues" when you skip a meal or snack is a slippery slope.

Hunger cues can also be suppressed by high levels of activity[xiii], which is ironic since that's when we need to fuel the most. Stress can also impact how hungry you feel. So, for high school and college-aged athletes, while we want you to tune into your feelings, we don't want you to trust them entirely.

Even if you don't struggle with restriction, it may take a while to fully hone your ability to tune into your hunger cues, so remember: It's better to fuel than to not fuel!

We like to think about hunger cues as an addition to eating on a relatively stable schedule. What we mean by that is that hunger cues should rarely be used to skip a meal or a snack—instead, use them to *add* a meal or a snack. The more regular your eating schedule is, the more likely you are to feel good, healthy hunger cues.

You may also find that you're feeling uncomfortably full after every meal. In that case, zoom out and look at how you're eating, not just what you're eating. Are you eating while you rush between classes, eating as fast as you can in order to get to the next thing? Unfortunately, how you eat can impact your digestion as much as what you eat. Slow down and give your body a chance to enjoy the food!

You might be wondering why we don't like the idea of getting uncomfortably full, considering we've spent this whole book telling you to eat more. Well, that's because when we're too full from a meal to have our snack a couple hours later, we miss that snack or maybe skip an entire meal, and then we either end up in that deficit and underfueled state or we overeat later in the day and the cycle begins again.

Hunger cues help us eat the right amount: If you are an individual who struggles with overeating to the point of feeling overly full later in the day, you may notice that you're caught in a cycle. You're too full, then you feel a little sick going to bed, then you skip breakfast, then you're starving again by the afternoon, and it just kind of becomes this perpetual pattern.

For most athletes, stick to eating three meals and two snacks during the day. The amount you eat can vary based on those hunger cues, but stick to the schedule.

Figuring out your optimal strategies for good digestion can take time, but it's possible. If you feel like you've tried everything and still can't quite get it dialed in, though, it's a good idea to seek professional help from a registered dietitian who specializes in working with athletes. There may be an underlying issue that you're not going to be able to solve alone!

THE IMPORTANT EXTRAS

NUTRITION MATTERS—BUT there are a lot of factors at play in your body. Things like how much or how well you sleep can impact how easily you're able to digest and utilize the fuel that you're taking in. Your hormones will fluctuate, which can change how you feel and how your gut reacts to different foods. And we're also going to dig into some nutrition trends that are doing more harm than good.

11 / SLEEP 101

No, sleep isn't a nutrient—but it might as well be for how important it is to your nutrition! Basically, without sleep, the stuff you eat simply isn't as effective for helping your body. Sleep is key when it comes to your body being able to digest and actually use the nutrients that you've taken in during the day to perform a number of key processes to restore and prepare your body for the day ahead. These processes include repairing, rebuilding and building new muscle, keeping your immune system strong, and improving your brain function. Sleep also significantly impacts your performance by improving reaction time, speeding muscle recovery, lowering injury risk, improving metabolic function, and improving cognitive function. It's the key to both mental and physical health. It improves mood and reduces stress. It regulates your hormones, including growth hormones. Sleep supports better decision-making, focus and learning abilities. And that doesn't just apply to school. In your sport, you need to learn different aspects, tactics and plays, and execute on them.

Basically, it can't be overstated how important sleep is: You can eat the 'perfect' diet and follow a training plan to the letter, but if you're not getting enough sleep, nothing is going to work. Inadequate sleep is going to hinder the ability to learn new skills, make quick decisions and recover effectively.

Sleep is critical for younger athletes in particular, which is why we decided to include it in this book. It's the only time during the day when most of us are actually giving our bodies a break, and it's key to great sport performance on both race day and in the long term.

Most teenagers require eight to ten hours of sleep per night to function optimally[i]—yes, that's more than the seven to nine typically recommended for adults. And for athletes, the higher end of that spectrum tends to be the preferred amount of sleep, since you're doing so much work and require so much more recovery. (Remember: This number refers to the hours you're asleep, not the hours you're lying in bed, so if it takes you a while to fall asleep, you need an even earlier bedtime!)

But to access this magic nutrient—trust us, sleep is better than any supplement on the market!—you may need to do some work.

Ironically, despite needing more sleep, athletes are at a higher risk for sleep problems due to their lifestyle. Athletes tend to have early morning and late night practices, and student athletes are juggling school work with training and maybe trying to have a social life... Logistically, it's hard to get enough sleep, and even harder to get good quality sleep.

You may have heard that napping or 'banking sleep'(sleeping more on weekends when you have time) isn't good for your sleep hygiene and won't actually help you. But research[ii] has shown that for younger athletes, sleep banking and naps are actually *incredibly* helpful, so consider this your approval note for sleeping in on Sunday. Yes, you should strive for eight to ten hours of sleep every night. But from Monday to Friday, if you truly only can carve out time for seven, get that ten or even eleven hours on Friday and Saturday nights whenever possible, and sneak in a few naps[iii] when you can.

There's a reason we talked about not wanting to overdo the caffeine back in Chapter 7. If you are waking up in need of caffeine and you are relying on it throughout the day to stay awake and alert, this is a huge red flag that something is wrong. Often, it's a combination of not fueling enough and not sleeping enough. Using caffeine to keep you going throughout the day is like trying to use a Bandaid to fix a broken leg. We need to zoom out and really address a few foundational things, rather than just slapping a caffeine Bandaid on the problem. And that starts with fixing our sleep.

The other diet myth we want to debunk for you when it comes to sleep is the one that says you shouldn't eat for a few hours before going to bed. Yes, for sedentary adults who tend to over-consume calories, this is a good rule. But for a young athlete, this rule does not exist. Consider this your permission slip to eat before bed. For you, eating is more important than the potential for minor sleep disruption, and it won't hurt your metabolism. If anything, it will help you. Eating enough is far more important than not eating past eight o'clock, especially for athletes who are training in the afternoon or evening.

That being said, your bedtime snack can be selected to optimize for sleep rather than a tossing-and-turning indigestion-fest overnight. A glass of chocolate milk (or a hot chocolate!) can be a perfect easy protein and carb-rich snack that actually promotes sleep. A bowl of cereal or oatmeal is great. Toast with peanut butter and jam? For sure. Basically, if you'd eat it for breakfast before a training session or a race, it's a good bedtime snack.

Skip greasy, fried, fatty options, since these tend to leave you tossing and turning—and of course, skip anything caffeinated. (Again, our caveat: If you had a late training session and the only option in the fridge is leftover pizza, go ahead and eat the slice. You'll still sleep better eating pizza compared to going to bed hungry.)

Finally, set yourself up for success with the time you do have to spend in bed by optimizing your bedroom for sleep: Think cold, dark and quiet. Develop a wind-down routine that helps you feel ready to go to sleep, like reading, drinking a cup of herbal tea, or watching a relaxing show. Avoid things that will keep you up, like doomscrolling or watching horror movies. And keep track of the changes you make by noting them in a training log or sleep journal: You'll start to learn what works to help you sleep better, and what habits are keeping you awake at night.

Getting your sleep right is one of the biggest positive changes that you can make, and like drinking enough water, the best part is that it's free.

12 / UNDERSTAND YOUR HORMONES

Ahh, hormones. Can't live without them, but they can make life a major pain sometimes. We're not going too in-depth on hormones, since entire books are written about just that topic. But we did want to give you an overview, since hormones can seriously impact your ability to train and perform at a high level when something is off, and can potentially affect how you should approach your fueling. As a young female athlete, your hormones are hugely important—ignore at your peril.

For young women athletes, you're not just contending with a consistent baseline of hormones: Your body is changing throughout the month thanks to your menstrual cycle. The menstrual cycle is the cycle of building up the lining in your uterus and, assuming you're not pregnant, shedding it (that part is when you actually get your period) every 21 to 38 days. Having a regular menstrual cycle is a good thing! When you first get your period, it may be irregular for the first couple of years, but it should eventually become more regular. During the menstrual cycle, your body goes through four phases—menstruation, the follicular phase, ovulation, and the luteal phase—and during each, the hormones in your body will be working in different ways.

Hormones in general tend to get a bad rap: They're often blamed for causing problems, but the reality is that when they're in balance, they're helping you thrive. So let's dig into the key ones you should know about before we talk about how to contend with things like birth control or hormones that seem out of whack.

Estrogen is a necessary hormone when it comes to maintaining good reproductive health—which isn't just something you need if you want to get pregnant, it's important for overall health as well. Estrogen levels are going to naturally fluctuate a bit during your menstrual cycle, but in general, a healthy body won't leave a healthy estrogen range. Too much is bad, too little is bad.

Estrogen also impacts blood cholesterol levels, blood sugar levels, bone mass and muscle mass[i]. When we don't have enough estrogen, this can lead to that bone loss and potentially lead to a stress fracture. So if we see stress fractures and bone stress injuries, we often look at estrogen levels to see what's going on.

Progesterone is another key hormone that's similar to estrogen: It regulates your menstrual cycle, impacts bone mass, and is important for muscle strength, recovery as well as regulating body temperature, which fluctuates slightly throughout the menstrual cycle[ii].

And then there's **testosterone**—yep, it's not just for men! We don't have as much as men, but we do have it and it's very important, especially for athletes. It's key for maintaining muscle mass and lean body mass[iii]. And good news, normally, our bodies are able to regulate it just fine, as long as we're eating enough.

The same is true of **cortisol**, often referred to as the stress hormone. It's a naturally occurring hormone that's healthy in the right amount, problematic if it gets too low or too high. Your cortisol levels are generally at their highest in the morning, dropping throughout the day so you're ready to sleep at night. Like the other hormones we mentioned here, the best way to keep cortisol regulated, in addition to keeping your stress levels low-to-moderate, is to be eating enough, sleeping enough and not overdoing the training.

As women go through puberty, estrogen and progesterone levels naturally rise, and this is what leads to breast development and changes in body composition in addition to getting a period. For athletes, this change can feel scary and stressful, and many are tempted to try to stop it altogether. But it's a positive thing!

Unfortunately, low estrogen or progesterone[iv] can happen purposely *or* accidentally. Big factors that are going to lower both include over-exercising and underfueling[v]. (More on that in the next chapter.)

It's important to understand that if you try to stop puberty or the typical weight gain that comes with it, you're hurting those systems as well. By delaying the onset of puberty by underfueling and making it impossible for your body to produce the hormones it needs to develop, whether intentionally or unintentionally, you're going to have an increased risk for bone injuries[vi], particularly stress fractures. In your teens and early twenties, you're in a critical growth period, so if you are not giving the body all the resources it needs to grow during that time, you're setting yourself up for a shorter career and potential for poor bone health throughout your life. Remember, women tend to peak later than men: You have until your late thirties to hit your stride in your sport (possibly even longer) so avoid taking shortcuts in your teens and early twenties.

To make a long story short: Low energy availability—not having enough fuel on board to support the work you're doing—suppresses all of your primary hormones that we just mentioned[vii], making it impossible for them to do all the good stuff that they do. From negatively impacting your performance right now to increasing your risk of stress fractures in the near future to even impairing your reproductive function in both short-term and long-term, when hormones aren't working right, your body isn't working right.

So, how do you know your hormones are working for you? The number one sign of good hormone health is getting a regular period (between 21 and 35 day cycles that include two to seven days of bleeding)[viii]. Not getting your period—amenorrhea—is a sign that something isn't right with your hormones, and puts you at much higher risk of athletic injury as well as decreased performance.

But periods as an indicator of good hormone health are tricky. First of all, athletes who recently got their period may take a couple of years before their cycle is regular, so this isn't a great indicator. And for young women who are using hormonal birth control, whether the birth control pill, a hormonal IUD or some other hormone-based type of birth control[ix], it can be hard to tell if your hormones are in tip-top shape since you're artificially impacting them and the bleed that you get on hormonal birth control isn't a true period. Even a copper IUD that doesn't contain hormones can sometimes cause excessive bleeding, which can also make it hard to tell if you're menstruating in a way that is optimally healthy for your body.

The downside of birth control is that it makes it hard to tell if our cycle is regular, since on the birth control pill (often referred to as 'The Pill'), the breakthrough bleed you have in week four isn't actually your period. Similarly, with a hormonal IUD, it's entirely possible you won't have any bleeding at all. Does that mean you're not getting a period and something is wrong? Not necessarily. What this *does* mean for you is that you won't get the warning sign of a missed or irregular period.

Yes, a missed or irregular period is one of the best early warning signs for low energy availability. But not having it as a potential symptom—either because your period is still irregular because it started recently or because you're on hormonal birth control—means you need to pay more attention to how you're feeling, and be on the lookout for other symptoms like fatigue, decreased performance and gut issues.

If you're put on birth control to 'bring back' your period, beware —especially as an athlete, this can mask symptoms of underfueling. Remember, the 'period' you get on the birth control pill is a breakthrough bleed, not a true period, so it can make it seem as though you're 'fixed' but the underlying issues aren't addressed at all. The

Pill does not impact the underlying problem of energy deficiency. It also will not fix the associated declines in bone density and other negative health outcomes that come from underfueling. The birth control pill can also deplete certain micronutrients[x], which can add to issues of iron deficiency that are common in young women, and can also elevate our cortisol levels.

Now, it's worth mentioning that birth control is obviously extremely helpful and important! But while we are firm believers in your right to use birth control, it is important to understand the trade-offs that each method carries, and be aware that the bleed you get on the birth control pill is not an indicator of health.

Speaking of birth control, get ready for a teeny tiny sex talk: At your age (assuming you're in your late teens or twenties), you *should* have a sex drive. Obviously, there are exceptions here, whether due to your orientation if you identify as asexual, due to some underlying health issue that you're already aware of, due to certain medications, or due to trauma or mental health issues. But if you're generally in good health mentally and physically and don't consider yourself asexual, having interest in sex is both normal and a good sign of hormonal health. I consider—and research supports that—low or no sex drive, especially if it's recently dropped, to be a red flag that something is going on[xi].

On the note of your period, assuming that you're getting one, it's become very trendy to train according to where you are in your cycle[xii]. It's made a lot of headlines in recent years. So, is it worth doing? Not for a serious athlete. There are so many factors that impact training, and where you are in your cycle is just a small piece of the overall puzzle. It doesn't make sense to shift your training to match your phase when there are so many other factors you could train around as well—not to mention, as a serious athlete, you don't get to pick where race day or competitions fall in your cycle.

Yes, some athletes are very much impacted by their cycle[xiii,xiv], due to things like premenstrual syndrome (PMS) or a painful period, but in general, our periods shouldn't be a major issue or impact our training. And if you are impacted enough by PMS or a painful period that it regularly affects your training, definitely talk to your doctor, because that isn't normal and it isn't something you should have to put up with.

The only part of your cycle you should use as a cue to change things up is listening to what your body is craving, since in different phases, you may need or want more carbohydrates. Lean in during those times!

It can also be helpful to track your cycle and how it impacts training and performance—not so you can shift your training to work better with your period, but so that you can learn more about how your body works and what to expect from it—and particularly, when to give yourself some grace. You may find that at certain times in your cycle, you need a bit more recovery time and some extra sleep. That's useful information, since if you know you have a big competition around that point in your cycle, you can make sure you plan out extra hours in bed.

To grab our free PDF printout of our easy hormone tracker, head to StrongGirlPublishing.com/power-up for all the free resources and bonus material!

Underfueling and overtraining can impact all of your hormones, but here's the final, trickier piece of the puzzle to be aware of: *So can stress.* That's right, having final exams, a fight with a friend, and a major competition in the same week can cause serious hormonal havoc. Stress can disrupt different aspects of our hormones, starting with an overproduction of cortisol, which can impact mood regulation and brain function. And when combined with underfueling and overtraining, stress is even harder on the body[xv].

All of the body systems work together—your emotional and physical health are closely linked, and hormones are sort of the middle man that goes between the two, causing the most disruption. But luckily, the best defense is to fuel enough, sleep enough, and train appropriately. (We know it's not as simple as it sounds, but it is possible!)

If you suspect something is out of whack with your menstrual cycle, you should talk to your doctor and potentially get your hormones tested. However, the treatment plan for low hormones is essentially doing what we recommend in this book: Eat enough, especially in and around training, and make sure that you're not overtraining. You can start doing that right now!

13 / WHAT HAPPENS WHEN YOU UNDERFUEL?

TRIGGER WARNING: *This section discusses eating disorders, restrictive eating, and disordered eating*

We've mentioned underfueling and how it can lead to issues with performance and overall health throughout the book, but it deserves its own chapter since it can go from something as simple as feeling bad during practice because you missed lunch to something that can potentially derail your entire athletic career. Underfueling has a lot of different names and acronyms, and it can be really confusing to navigate, especially as a young woman athlete who is out there just trying her best—and yet is still struggling. Relative Energy Deficiency in Sport (often abbreviated as RED-s and REDs), Low Energy Availability (LEA), and the still-mentioned but now-defunct Female Athlete Triad are all essentially the same thing: the effects of being chronically underfueled, often overtrained, or a combination of both[i]. And the short version of this chapter is that you want to avoid these issues at all costs, especially as a female athlete.

A key sign that you're underfueling and/or not eating enough carbohydrates is fatigue, both in and out of training[ii]. Carbohydrates provide energy for the body, so without them, your battery is essentially being drained. You may also find that you have a hard time concentrating, experience mood swings, even get headaches, and generally have poor sleep (you know when you wake up after a long time in bed and you just do not feel rested or recovered). School assignments and things that never used to stress you out may start to make your brain feel fuzzy or overwhelmed. Physically, you may notice that you're more bloated and constipated. You'll likely notice that your performance in your sport is going down, and you're struggling to recover after workouts. You just won't have the same 'oomf' that you used to, that extra bit that helps you sprint to the finish line. You may notice that you're more anxious than usual, or struggle to find joy in things you used to love. You're missing that pep in your step.

A simplified way to think about it is to think of LEA as the short-term consequences and REDs as the long-term consequences of underfueling[iii]. LEA happens when the body doesn't have enough energy to meet its needs in a particular workout. It can occur when an athlete's overall intake is too low and or they expend too much energy through exercise. And when it happens often enough and for a prolonged period of time, you end up in REDs.

REDs can be challenging to diagnose, as it requires a comprehensive evaluation by an expert like a physician who specializes in sports medicine[iv]. To add another layer to this, the symptoms of overtraining syndrome and REDs have a lot of overlap. But in general, when your energy intake and energy expenditure do not match up, when you're not consuming enough food overall energy to meet the energy demands of training and daily life, it catches up with you and the consequences can be not just short-term, but also impact your life in sport and health in the long haul.

Unfortunately, we tend to miss the early signs of REDs and only start to pay attention to it when our performance in our sport is impacted. But by the time we start noticing the decline in athletic performance, we may already be dealing with some of the less-obvious but more detrimental long-term issues like a reduction in bone mineral density[v,vi]. That's why one of the most obvious signs of

REDs is when an athlete gets a stress fracture, especially if it's in an area that isn't being loaded during sport. We see a lot of hip, femur and sacrum stress reactions and fractures from REDs, though other stress fractures can certainly be related to REDs[vii]. And as we mentioned in the hormone chapter, a menstrual cycle that's irregular or suddenly stops (amenorrhea) is a primary indicator of REDs. However, because often young athletes don't yet have fully regular cycles or may be on birth control that prevents them from knowing if their hormones are balanced, a period (or lack thereof) isn't always a great indicator of REDs. Unfortunately, a lot of doctors still use the period as a primary indicator and don't look beyond that, so if you are on birth control or know your period is always irregular, make sure you're advocating hard for yourself and support for a diagnosis.

If you have Functional Hypothalamic Amenorrhea (FHA), the fancy way of saying you aren't getting your period due to overtraining/underfueling/stress, you'll be more susceptible to getting sick and your cardiovascular health can be impacted[viii]. You may have an iron deficiency, your growth and development—even height!—can be impaired. It can cause gut issues because it slows down your metabolism and messes with your digestion, and it can impact your sleep. And it can definitely impact your mental health and your mental well being, whether it's feeling anxious, feeling depressed, or feeling flat. You may have constant brain fog[ix]. Short version: It's going to impact every system in your body in a negative way.

And here's the scary thing: Often, athletes aren't trying to lose weight or underfuel intentionally[x]. Yes, disordered eating and eating disorders are distressingly common for young women athletes[xi]. And if you suspect that you're dealing with one of those issues, please talk to someone and get help! But LEA and REDs are not always related to eating disorders or disordered eating, and we athletes do a huge disservice when we assume that they're automatically linked. In fact, even body weight isn't a great indicator for LEA or REDs[xii].

Especially for busy student athletes, it can be hard to eat enough, and to eat *regularly* enough, to meet your body's massive energy demands. Maybe you're an athlete on scholarship or a tight budget, which can make it challenging to eat when the dining hall is closed or if you cannot find low-priced, nutrient-dense snacks. You're likely not intending to underfuel. It's just the way your schedule is. If you're in school, working and training, that essentially means that you have three full-time jobs. But eating needs to be your fourth shift!

Unfortunately, if you end up in a state of LEA, even unintentionally, you may feel like it's your fault, like you've done something wrong. You haven't. You just didn't know. Too often, we end up with feelings of shame around issues like this, and those feelings prevent us from getting the help that we actually need. That's why we wrote this book: **to help normalize eating more, eating enough and eating to support our bodies.**

REDs is undoubtedly a very serious issue for athletes, and we'll be blunt here, there are some athletes who never manage to fully recover from it, or who deal with issues related to it for decades after. But many athletes are able to make a full recovery and continue on to long careers in sport.

The biggest part of recovery is going to be increasing overall energy intake. Oftentimes, we also benefit from modifications to training and exercise for a short period, especially if injury or illness is occurring. If it's a critical situation, there's usually a longer duration with no exercise until we start to see progress in the right direction. But for most athletes, we don't need to stop our sport entirely. We can find a happy medium with exercise, because the mental and physical benefits of sport, plus the social connections with our teammates, often outweigh the concerns.

And yes: There may be some weight gain involved as you come out of REDs and LEA[xiii]. It's normal and expected—and almost always healthy and necessary. Your body will come to the weight where it's healthiest if you're fueling and training in balance. And if you're concerned about abrupt weight gain as you start to work on your fueling, check in with a doctor or dietitian to help you find the right balance for you.

Finally, a question that athletes often have is whether or not REDs or LEA can happen to an athlete who is in a bigger body[xiv]. Yes, absolutely. You do not have to be a thin white girl to struggle with REDs, despite the fact that 'thin and white' tends to be how the media portrays it. You may have noticed we didn't include weight loss as a symptom of REDs. In fact, it may sound impossible, but weight gain sometimes can be an outcome of LEA and REDs thanks to the way both mess with your metabolism!

In fact, in my clinical practice, about 90 percent of the people I work with are women. And almost all of them come to me with the same problem: They're training for a big race like a marathon or Ironman, and yet, they're gaining weight. It's rarely because they're not exercising enough or eating too much. It's almost always because they're underfueling. When you underfuel, your body goes haywire. Those hormones that control your metabolism don't react the way that they should. Your body is holding on to everything—hence the bloating and constipation we mentioned as symptoms. So, no, REDs doesn't automatically make you 'thinner.'

REDs also does not discriminate. It can happen at any time of life, any body shape and size. And yes, it tends[xv] to be more prevalent in sports where weight is a concern, either due to weight classes (like rowing or boxing) or sports where a smaller body is generally considered to be 'better' (like distance running or gymnastics). But unintentional underfueling can happen in any sport—especially for busy student athletes who don't have easy access to food throughout the day.

If you believe that you're dealing with LEA or REDs, it's important to talk to your coach, doctor or dietitian as soon as possible to come up with a plan to work your way back to your healthiest self. The earlier you can catch signs of chronic underfueling, the better your chance for a full recovery—the best thing you can do as an athlete is become more self-aware and catch these things before they become major problems.

WHAT ABOUT WEIGHT LOSS?

You didn't think we'd completely skip over talking about weight loss, did you? Heck, no. (Though it was tempting, because this subject is seriously tricky.) But we didn't want to insult your intelligence or do you a disservice by pretending that young women athletes aren't thinking about if they should lose weight, how to lose weight, or when to lose weight.

Short version: If you're reading this book, weight loss likely shouldn't be a goal for you[xvi]. At your age—assuming you're under 27—we want you to get the idea of 'weight loss' out of your head entirely, especially in terms of rapid weight loss or even that cliche of 'losing one pound per week' being the 'healthy amount.' At your age, as your body—hormones, bones, brain and everything else—is still going through massive changes, you're not in a good position to focus on weight loss. Yes, you might lose weight with some of the recommendations we're going to talk about, but it should be a very long-term game, not a short-term 'how low can I go?'

Maybe you saw a teammate drop 15 pounds and crush it last season, or you noticed that your times got slower when you put on 10 pounds after hitting puberty. This is the short term lie that the scale tells you: The lie that losing weight is how you get better/faster/stronger. The longer-term view (even a year or two out) is much different: Typically, those rapid weight losses catch up to athletes and cause issues like injury and illness[xvii]. Weight gain, especially during this phase of life, can come with short-term slow downs in speed, but almost always will result in eventual improved performance. But patience is hard!

If you are thinking about losing weight, please talk to a doctor and/or dietitian rather than trying to do it on your own.

The reality is that if you're eating well and fueling your training, your body will come to settle at the weight that is healthiest and most optimal for you. That's right, that idea that there is one optimal weight or body composition is a myth. Each and everyone of us has its own optimal weight and body composition. And if you're an athlete, you likely want to perform at your best. So what works for your teammate might not work for you. If a body is underfed and stressed out, that is not a body that can be expected to perform well... Regardless of what the scale says.

As a young female athlete, you're trying to compete at your highest level now and build a career that could last well into your thirties and early forties. Trying to force your body to lose or gain weight at will is a nearly guaranteed way to ensure that your career will be shorter than you'd like it to be.

To this end, we're big fans of chucking the scale. Even at the doctor or dietitian's office, we suggest asking to not be told the number. The number on the scale shouldn't be scary, but the fact is that most of us are subconsciously or consciously affected by it in a way that just is not useful. And for young women, it's nearly impossible to have a healthy relationship with a number on the scale, especially because it's frankly an ever-changing number—your weight can easily change up to five pounds per day and will change throughout your menstrual cycle. Your scale weight even depends on whether or not you've pooped this morning or not!

So put it away. Take away its power. If we don't even give the scale the opportunity to define our worth and our abilities, then we're getting ahead of the game. If we can keep that out of the picture, then we can really lean into actual indicators of health and performance and how we're supporting our bodies. We can start to spot the connection between eating a bedtime snack and feeling stronger and faster in swim practice in the morning. This is much more helpful than getting on the scale and seeing a number that's two pounds higher than usual, then deciding to skip the snack and having your performance suffer. Rather than making choices driven by a number on the scale, we can make choices driven by our performance, our energy levels, our sleep, et cetera.

Here's the ultimate irony: Of all of the women we spoke to in working on this book, almost all of them said the same thing. They wished they had focused less on their weight as young athletes. Not only that, but they found that years later, when they stopped stressing about the scale and eating 'perfectly,' they ended up being their fittest, strongest selves because they stopped restricting and stopped trying to fight their bodies.

Sometimes, you need to let go of the idea of the 'ideal weight' or the 'perfect body' to let your body get to where it wants to be—and often, the results will surprise you (in a good way!).

LET'S STOP TALKING ABOUT WEIGHT AND BODY COMPOSITION AT PRACTICE

If your coach mentions weight on a regular basis, even if it doesn't trigger you, consider this your sign to speak up and ask them to stop. A focus on weight or body composition, whether it's intentional or not, creates an unhealthy and toxic training environment[xviii].

Coaches can sometimes be a bit old-school in their thinking and the way that they phrase things. They may still believe the outdated idea that being a lighter weight or having a lower body composition is automatically 'better.' We know that things like 'racing weight' aren't actually valid, especially for young athletes. We know that lighter doesn't always mean faster. We know that athletes need to eat enough, not compete to see who can eat the least.

But unfortunately, coaches often receive zero nutrition training, and are sharing often-outdated and inaccurate information[xix]. Even coaches trying to keep up with the best nutrition advice may find themselves awash in misinformation/disinformation! It's usually not purposeful, but we've heard one too many coaches talking about 'no ice cream until the offseason' and similar comments that seem to advocate for restrictive eating habits. (*Every* season is ice cream season.)

Advocate for yourself and your teammates: Ask the coach to stop talking about weight and to bring in a dietitian to speak to the team if you feel like the team could benefit from some third-party wisdom.

14 / WHAT'S THE DEAL WITH SUPPLEMENTS?

As a young athlete, you may notice that a lot of your teammates or other people you follow on social media are using supplements—pills, powders, and even IV bags with micronutrients, adaptogens, and a whole host of other maybe helpful, maybe harmful stuff. As we're writing this, it's impossible to scroll any social media or women's health-oriented website without seeing a powder or pill being marketed to us. Supplements can include anything from a multivitamin to protein powder, and even sports drinks and gels fall into this category. For young athletes especially, there are a lot of things you need to know about supplements before just hitting 'buy now' on Amazon, or filling your cart at the local pharmacy.

In this chapter, we're not talking about the nutrients themselves—head back to the nutrient chapters for that! We're talking strictly about these nutrients in a supplement form: Think protein powder instead of a chicken breast or calcium instead of milk. We'll get into a few of the supplements that are most commonly used/asked about by athletes, but first, let's chat about a few general caveats and things to know about supplements.

You should always focus on what you can get from your food first. Supplements are just that: *supplemental*. Meaning *extra*. That means you shouldn't substitute a greens powder for eating your vegetables, have protein powder instead of a meal that actually contains protein, something like chicken or tofu, or take any micronutrient like calcium or vitamin C in pill form rather than getting these nutrients from a food source. Yes, there are cases where supplements can be helpful, but in general, you should get almost all of your nutrient needs from food. This is just a good, smart, budget-friendly habit to get into.

With supplements, think short term, not full-time. As a dietitian, I do recommend supplements to clients sometimes, but it's always with a short term view. We'll add a certain vitamin or mineral based on bloodwork in order to bring that level up or address a need, but we'll retest after a few months. The goal is always to stop using any supplement, not to stay on the same regimen forever.

Always look for third party 'certified for sport' labels when you are choosing a supplement. If you have any goals of becoming a pro athlete or you're currently a collegiate athlete, you'll be subject to testing from your country's anti-doping organization. Supplements that aren't third party tested and certified can sometimes contain banned ingredients (purposefully or not). And yes, getting a protein powder that's labeled NSF Certified for Sport of Informed Choice is likely more expensive than the bargain brand at Walmart, but it's worth it. And not just for athletes who may get tested: A shocking percentage of supplements that aren't third-party tested have the strong potential to be harmful due to the number of unregulated ingredients that can sneak in there[i,ii]. Especially for young athletes, these unregulated supplements can contain unsafe and potentially harmful ingredients that can mess with your hormones and your overall health.

These third-party certified supplements tend to be more expensive and require more research on your part, but that's actually a positive, since it forces you to get clear on what you actually need rather than just grabbing bottles off the shelf. If the supplement actually matters enough to you that you want to use it, it *should* come at a cost.

If the high-quality protein powder is out of your budget, swap to tofu or yogurt instead.

At the end of the day, we aren't anti-supplement. But a supplement should not be a main character in our nutrition story. At best, they should be the witty best friend who occasionally pops up when our heroine (that's you) needs something a little extra. Here's what you need to know about the supplements we see most commonly recommended for young women athletes:

IRON

Young women especially are often told[iii] that "because you're a female athlete, you almost certainly will have low iron and you're going to have to take an iron supplement." But simply taking an iron supplement without any testing or considerations of your current fueling/training status isn't the right answer[iv]. You should not be looking at an iron supplement as a long-term solution to low iron. Furthermore, if you actually have low iron, that's not something that's "just a fact of life for female athletes," no matter what your coach says. That's an outdated perspective. Low iron means that there's likely something else going on or a shift in your diet that actually needs to be addressed.

If you need to take iron temporarily, that's one thing. But it's a Bandaid solution—it'll work for a while, but it's not a long term way to keep your iron levels in check[v,vi]. There are a number of factors that can impact your iron levels and your iron status[vii]. Obviously, if you're not eating enough iron-rich foods, your iron may be low. But if you're not eating enough in general, your iron may be low even if you're having an iron-rich steak every night. There are a lot of other micronutrients that are involved in the iron transport process—getting the iron where it needs to go,—and we often see the iron deficiency because an athlete is not getting enough of those supportive nutrients so that the iron can properly transport itself. For many athletes, low iron isn't from low iron content in food, it's from that overall underfueling[viii,ix].

Overtraining can also cause low iron because consistent inflammation from that training can inhibit the iron absorption process[x]. So if we're training hard six or seven days a week, not getting enough rest and not letting those inflammation levels come down, your iron stores drop.

As you can guess, taking an iron supplement doesn't solve for underfueling or overtraining. Sure, it can correct your iron levels temporarily. But it's not a long term fix for the underlying issues, and those issues will just present in other ways... Plus, the iron may be in your blood from a supplement, but if underfueling or overtraining is the cause of your low iron, the iron isn't going to be used properly. It's going to build up in the bloodstream, which then can also be harmful. Ironically, too much iron in the bloodstream can cause the same symptoms as low iron, like shortness of breath, fatigue, joint pain, and muscle weakness[xi]. It's not something that can quickly be fixed.

For more on iron, head back to the Micronutrients chapter on page 27.

PROTEIN POWDER

Protein is important, and can be difficult to get in whole food form if you're an athlete who is always on the go. But protein powder isn't my preferred protein source. I'd rather see athletes drinking a chocolate milk or having a more satisfying snack, especially younger athletes.

However, if you find a brand that is third-party tested and certified for sport, protein powder can be useful to have on hand for times where you just don't have time post-workout for a full meal. But it shouldn't be something you rely on all the time. It can absolutely be a tool in your toolbox, but not the only option.

We don't want to rely on protein powder, because when we eat whole foods, we're getting so much more than just protein. We're getting a lot of other micronutrients that we need in small quantities from the food itself. Protein powder, especially protein powder that is third party certified, also tends to be pricey—so don't feel like you need to have it on hand.

For more on protein, head back to the Protein chapter on page 13.

CAFFEINE/PRE-WORKOUT SUPPLEMENTS

We've already discussed caffeine in Chapter 7 on Pre-Workout Fueling, but it's worth mentioning here since it's arguably the most common supplement that athletes use. And yes, it is a supplement. While no one is judging you if you have a second cup of coffee, caffeine is considered a supplement, and yes, in high quantities, it's actually a *banned* supplement if you're competing in the NCAA[xii] as a collegiate athlete. Be wary of energy drinks that contain caffeine, since often they contain five or more times the amount of caffeine found in a cup of coffee.

Quick reminder: For adults over 18, 400 milligrams of caffeine per day is the maximum amount recommended. If you're between 13 and 18, the American Academy of Pediatrics recommends under 100 milligrams of caffeine per day—about a cup of coffee. If you're under 12, definitely skip caffeine altogether!

Too much caffeine can a) be illegal for competition, but more importantly, b) can cause all kinds of negative side effects from jitters to headaches to a racing heart to even—in extreme cases—death[xiii]. It's pretty hard to perform at your best if you're playing volleyball or trying to swing a golf club with jittery hands. There are several instances of teens dying from taking in too much caffeine, sometimes in the form of caffeine pills, but there are cases where it's simply from drinking too many high caffeine drinks.

Too much caffeine can also impact sleep, which—as we already talked about in Chapter 11—can impact your ability to recover, making it easier for your body to end up in an overtraining/underfueling cycle.

For what to think about pre-workout instead, head back to the Pre-Workout chapter on page 45.

ALL-IN-ONE SUPPLEMENTS / MULTIVITAMINS

If it sounds too good to be true, it almost certainly is. All-in-one supplements that promise a blend of every vitamin, mineral, probiotic, adaptogen, etc. that you "need" aren't worth the spend. Especially for younger athletes, they don't make sense[xiv].

First, they tend to be expensive, especially if they are third party certified for sport—and if they aren't, you absolutely shouldn't go near them.

And second, they rarely contain enough of any one micronutrient to make them worth taking. Unfortunately, 'crop dusting' has become popular in supplements—companies have started using the tiniest amount of certain pricier ingredients in order to claim that they're added to the supplement, but the reality is they're in the mix in such a small concentration that they won't have any benefit.

Even multivitamins aren't recommended unless your doctor or dietitian has suggested one[xv]. A high-quality multivitamin can be a helpful tool, but it's not something that I'm going to recommend to everyone—too often, people use these multivitamins or all in one supplements in place of having a high quality nutrient dense diet. Additionally, depending on if you're using any supplement recommended by your doctor, a multivitamin may contain certain vitamins or minerals that actually interact negatively with the supplement you actually need.

HOW TO THINK ABOUT ANY OTHER SUPPLEMENT

Basically, any other supplement that you hear about should likely be skipped unless a doctor or dietitian specifically recommends it for you and has a good justification for why you need it. As a young athlete, you should be able to get everything you need from food, and supplements are just going to be expensive extras.

Rather than reaching for the hot new supplement, ask yourself: Am I eating enough? Am I getting enough micronutrients and macronutrients? Am I fueling my training and recovering adequately? Am I sleeping enough? These big rocks aren't as fun to post about on social media since they're a little boring, but they are more effective, less expensive, and generally safer than trying to solve a problem with a supplement on your own.

Unless you're a world champion in your sport and working with sports medicine doctors and dietitians who are trying to help you eke out that last two percent of performance capability, there is rarely a real need to add supplements to your routine. The average teen/early twenties female athlete shouldn't have supplements on her radar.

Finally, remember especially with 'hot new supplements' that are suddenly trending: Almost all sports science research is done on men[xvi], so for women of any age, how efficacious a supplement will be is almost always a question mark. On rare occasions, some supplement studies will be done on women as well, but very rarely young women who are still growing and developing. So remember, no matter how good a supplement sounds or claims to be, it has almost certainly not been tested for an athlete like you—and could cause more harm than good.

SHOULD I SUPPLEMENT?

Still wondering? Use this decision tree to help you determine if supplementation may be appropriate for you.

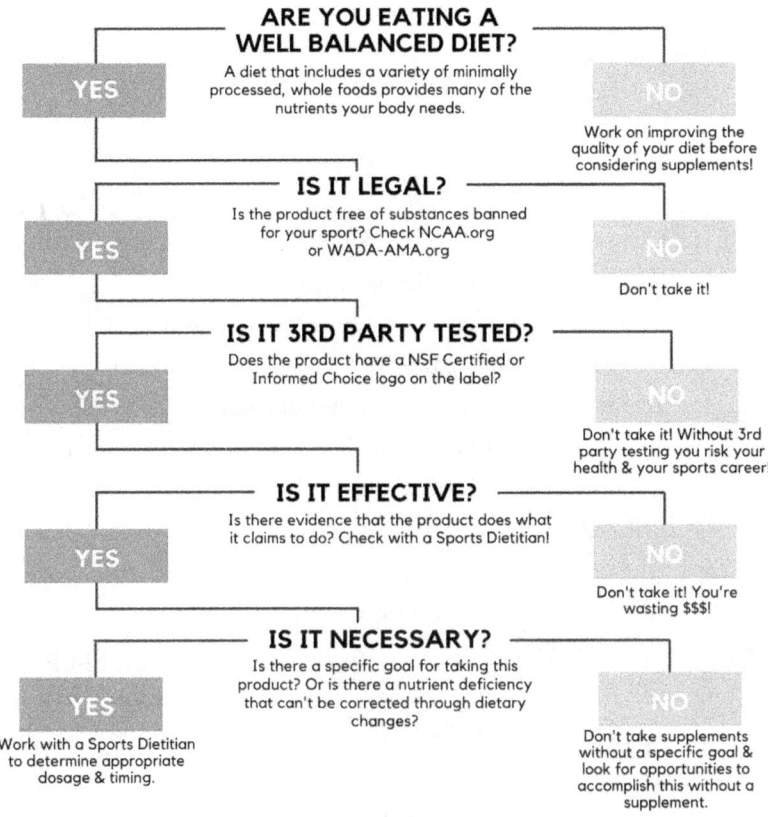

15 / WHAT NUTRITION TRENDS GET WRONG

IT SEEMS like every time you open your phone, there's another new nutrition trend on social media, or even a seemingly legit wellness website. But for young women athletes in particular, a lot of these trends can be incredibly unhelpful, if not downright dangerous because they are not rooted in evidenced-based research, but are often founded in pseudoscience (claims that sound scientific and are presented as fact but actually aren't based on real science) and mis/dis-information.

Often, these behaviors that are advertised as health-promoting may be applauded online based on number of likes or going viral, but in reality, they are very much disordered and have a strong potential to harm you. For example, intermittent fasting is one of the most widely accepted disordered behaviors I see in nutrition[i]—I talk to so many clients who are using it as a way to restrict without calling it restriction. I also see a lot of herbal supplements, enemas and laxatives being marketed as 'detoxifying' but clearly showcasing weight loss as the real desired result. Even using saunas can be a dangerous trend: I love saunas, I think they're great. We know that they can be health promoting, can reduce inflammation, and can be a great recovery tool[ii,iii]. But are you actually choosing to use the sauna every day because you think it's going to make you lose weight? And for the time-crunched athlete, we'll see more performance benefits from taking the time to—you guessed it—eat enough!

Whenever you're trying any wellness, nutrition or fitness trend, you have to pause and ask yourself *why* you're doing it. And be honest. Would you tell a doctor or dietitian that you're doing it? If it's about health or performance, you should have no problem telling a doctor or your coach. If you would be embarrassed or nervous to tell them, you're probably doing something that deep down, you know is harmful to your body in the long term.

Here are a few general trends to look out for and avoid at all costs.

SNEAKY RESTRICTIONS/RESTRICTING BEHAVIORS

Juice cleanses, no-carb or keto diets, intermittent fasting, longer-term fasting, elimination diets, anything calorie-cutting for weight loss or 'health' and, yes, even vegan diets can fall into the restrictive category.

Now, it does all depend on your why. For instance, in some cases, a dietitian may recommend an elimination diet if you're having specific issues[iv]. But no, you shouldn't try one at home on your own, especially if you intend to keep training at a high intensity at the same time. And yes, if you're passionate about animal rights, a vegan diet can absolutely be a healthy one. But if you're doing it strictly for health reasons or in order to avoid eating with your teammates or to eat fewer calories overall, think again.

The problem with these sneaky and seemingly societally approved versions of restrictive behavior is that—especially for athletes with a history of disordered eating or an eating disorder—at first glance, they seem healthy and helpful[v]. But in reality, they're allowing you to fall back into those restrictive behaviors that you know aren't serving you. These restrictions are a way to manipulate yourself and people around you into thinking that you're doing something healthy for yourself, but that is actually harmful behavior.

Any trend that tells you to restrict something is a red flag when it comes to nutrition and exercise and with having a healthy relationship with food, your body and exercise.

DETOXES OF ANY TYPE

Ahh, detoxes. They've been around for centuries and they *still* suck. In a single sentence, your body is always naturally detoxing itself, so you don't need to take a supplement to do that! Remember when we talked about poop back in Chapter 10? That's your body handling detox. Starving yourself, signing up for an expensive juice cleanse, taking pricey detox supplements or severely restricting the hours you're eating in a day—these are all just expensive and dangerous ways to ensure that your body can't do what it needs to do as a young athlete. (It should also go without saying that anything that claims to be a weight loss supplement is one that you should skip.)

First, let's talk toxins, AKA the thing you're detoxing *from*. There are different types of toxins that can harm the body[vi]: There are environmental toxins like air pollution, heavy metal toxicity and microbial toxins like mold, bacteria, and parasites. But toxins also include alcohol. I always like to drive that one home because it's the perfect example of the dose making the poison. Alcohol isn't a health drink regardless of how much you have, but a glass of wine is going to be relatively easy for most people to process and "detox" from. However, if you drink an entire bottle of wine, suddenly alcohol becomes a lot more toxic and potentially deadly. The same applies to most toxins: Living in a city like NYC is going to expose you to more air pollution than if you live in a small town in upstate New York[vii], but you're not necessarily going to become sick from the toxins in that city air—but you might if you live in a certain apartment with an unhealthy amount of fumes being pumped in.

The thought process behind a detox is that you're removing those aforementioned harmful substances, also known as toxins, from the body. It's a very popular concept, and understandably so. Wouldn't you love to believe that there's something in your gut that's limiting your playing capabilities, and that a certain pill or juice cleanse will cure it? That'd be nice... But there's very limited scientific evidence to support any type of detox's effectiveness outside of a hospital setting where a doctor has found that you have something that you need detoxing *from*.

Our bodies are really amazing things, and they can do detoxification on their own for most things. The liver, kidneys and even your skin are working together to help remove toxins from your body. Your kidneys and liver filter toxins out of the blood into your urine and waste, and then you go to the bathroom and remove those toxins. When you sweat, toxic products are removed through the skin via sweat.

Now, you can support your body's natural detoxification process, the same way you would do maintenance on your car to keep it running smoothly. You just need to support your elimination processes in a simple, natural way. That support looks like drinking enough water so that you're hydrated and therefore urinating and sweating at an appropriate rate. And because when we poop, our body is getting rid of toxins and things that we don't need in excess in our bodies, we want to be pooping regularly. That means making sure that you're eating enough, since underfueling can impact your digestive system. It also means eating a variety of high-fiber foods—all those fruits and vegetables!—because that's going to help you poop, along with adequate hydration. And sleep is when our body really does a lot of the detox work, so prioritizing enough sleep is also a way to promote your body's natural detoxification processes. And guess what? All of that is free. No weird pills, shakes, juices, or protocols required.

You can also control things like your drinking water: If you're worried about drinking from lead pipes because your house is older and may have lead pipes, you can use a water filter (like a Brita filter, and any fridge filter, as long as changed regularly) that pulls any heavy metals out of the water. We can't change our plumbing, but we can change our drinking water[viii].

Finally, coming back to the question we posed at the start of this chapter: What is your real 'why' for wanting to do a detox? The problem is not just the detox itself. It's also the fact that you think that you need to do a detox or a cleanse for some reason. Is that reason because you're having health issues that should indicate it's time to talk to your doctor? Or is it that you feel bloated after partying on the weekend and feel the urge to drop a couple of pounds quickly? Often, it's less about really thinking there's something you need to detox from and more about wanting to drop weight—and that's a problem.

ANYTHING CLAIMING TO GET RID OF 'BAD STUFF'

Detox supplements can also masquerade as supplements to help clear up things like bacteria or yeast overgrowth like SIBO (small intestinal bacterial overgrowth) or candida, parasites and worms, and any other 'gut distress causing critters.'[ix] If you suspect that you need some kind of support dealing with a bad gut bacteria situation, that is not something you should attempt to treat on your own. For starters, without testing, you don't know what's going on in your gut[x]—and you're more likely to harm the good gut bacteria living there versus getting rid of anything that shouldn't be!

This also comes back to the "why?" behind your urge to get rid of bacterial overgrowth, et cetera. Often, when clients really get honest about why they believed they had an issue with SIBO or a parasite (rarely the case) it was less about gut distress or pain and more about bloating or weight gain that they hoped would go away after "treating" the issue. Once again, the "why" is secretly weight loss-motivated.

If you genuinely think that something is wrong in your gut, you may very well be right—but no random supplement is going to fix it. You need to figure out what's going on. Always go to a medical provider who can test to see if you do need any supplemental help, because also a lot of those supplements and things being used in popular over the counter detox supplements can be very taxing on your liver. In fact, there are too many stories of people who have liver failure from taking supplements. And of course, you aren't even positive what you're getting! In most countries, including the US, supplements aren't regulated in the same way that food is, and the ones that claim to be detoxifying can do serious damage to your liver[xi].

"HEALTHIFIED" FOODS

How do you know you are being sold something that is healthified? When we say healthified, we're talking about foods/drinks/supplements that are making claims about how healthy and often 'clean' they are, but when you get into the nitty gritty of the ingredients list, you realize that it's more marketing claims than actual nutrition. And some of these foods are fine—but eating them may cause some gut distress, will likely be expensive, and may crowd out actually healthy foods from your diet.

Healthified foods include things like probiotic sodas, bars that are low-carb but packed with artificial sweeteners, protein powders and bars that have added fiber, even foods that are gluten-free or vegan but marketed as "healthy alternatives" despite being packed with added sugars and saturated fats. Foods like these are all commonly marketed to teens as being healthy, but the reality for an athletic young adult is that often, they aren't going to help you hit your performance goals.

For example, protein snacks that are high fiber usually have added inulin or chicory root, which doesn't really act like fiber from our foods—it's more likely to upset your stomach. Chicory root is a prebiotic fiber, so while it can be beneficial in some contexts, it can really alter someone's digestion and cause bloating and other gut issues like the urgent need to sprint from the pool to the bathroom.

If you love the prebiotic soda, that's fine. Just make sure you actually enjoy the taste and it doesn't bother your stomach—it's always worth pausing and reflecting on that, asking the question of whether you actually like something or if it's just been marketed to you really well.

FASTING/INTERMITTENT FASTING

Fasting and intermittent fasting—fasting for certain times of the day and only eating during a short window—fall into the restrictive category, but they're getting their own section here as well because they've become so popularized that they actually seem almost normal. But for young women athletes in particular, fasting or intermittent fasting can be incredibly detrimental[xii,xiii].

We need to make sure that we're eating enough to support our training, our school work, our growth, our development. So anything that we are doing to potentially restrict our energy intake is a big, big red flag. Our energy demands and needs are so high that if we create a short window where we're allowed to eat, we're making it nearly impossible to eat enough.

It can also have a very negative impact on female hormones, especially when you're in that reproductive development age: Fasting can impact our hormones negatively, which impacts your menstrual cycle. Fasting can also increase your cortisol levels, which can potentially increase blood sugar levels, disrupt thyroid function and cause fatigue, hunger, and inflammation.

Again, let's first dig into your "why." Fasting can be very tempting to do in the cases where you had a big weekend of partying, or you ate a lot of "bad food" over the weekend. We all have times where we overindulge—and again, this is where the "why" for fasting shifts from being health conscious to being weight loss focused. Notice when you suddenly are intrigued by the idea of fasting or intermittent fasting.

It's normal to have negative thoughts about your body and body image some days, especially with all the comparisons to ourselves with social media. But extremes like going on a fast are not the way to approach feeling more comfortable or feeling better in your body. Instead, think long term: doing the foundational things like hydrating, eating fruits and vegetables and whole grains and protein, balancing that performance plate out with those nourishing foods. Think about treating your body like your best friend.

The caveat to fasting is when fasting is being done for religious reasons: It's not easy to train while fasting for Ramadan, but if your religious beliefs dictate that you fast, it's entirely possible to do so. If this is the case, though, make sure your coach is aware of your current limitations, and if possible, talk to a dietitian to optimize the times when you are able to eat.

DO-IT-ALL SUPPLEMENTS / SUPPLEMENTS MEANT FOR LONG TERM USE

This trend is less about being potentially unhealthy and more about being potentially expensive and wasteful—but with some potential health issues in there too! There are a lot of supplements on the market now that are being touted by influencers and even mainstream media as being a do-it-all or all-in-one supplement that will improve, well, *everything*. These supplements are also typically marketed for long-term usage, meaning that you aren't just on them for three months to fix a shortcoming, you're taking them every day forever.

But they won't contain game-changing amounts of the ingredients they contain. This is known as "crop dusting." Even with certified, tested supplements, they don't need to list the amounts of each of the ingredients in the blend, so rarely do they include enough of any of the micronutrients or other additions like probiotics or adaptogens to be an effective dose for what you need. Additionally, sometimes these can interact with each other. For instance, in a daily multivitamin that contains both iron and calcium, the calcium inhibits the iron absorption—so you think that you're covering all of your nutritional bases, but you're actually taking a step backwards!

They can change your habits for the worse. If you think you're getting all of your major micronutrients from a single supplement, you may be less likely to eat nutrient-dense foods for the rest of the day because you assume you've checked all the boxes already.

Finally, they're expensive. Yes, some of these supplements are completely innocuous. They've been third-party certified and are safe for athletes to consume. But those supplements that are tested and certified tend to cost upwards of $75 to $100 per month, which is a lot when you're on a student budget. That can be a week of groceries! So no, you definitely don't need that all-in-one. Save the cash so you're not stressed when checking out at the grocery store next week.

As we said in Chapter 14, supplements should be short-term protocols, then reevaluated. Stop thinking of supplements as supplements, period. Instead, think of them as supplement protocols—and protocols have an end date. If you're taking a supplement, it's for a specific reason, for a specific duration, and you have a plan as to when you'll reevaluate if it's needed.

ADRENAL FATIGUE OR LEAKY GUT "SUPPORT"

It makes a lot of sense that young women athletes often assume that they're suffering from adrenal fatigue or leaky gut and seek solutions to these issues online, especially since most doctors will scoff when you mention either of them—typically unexplained fatigue and unexplained gut issues that just won't go away. While the symptoms of adrenal fatigue and leaky gut are real, adrenal fatigue and leaky gut are not medical diagnoses. In fact, adrenal fatigue and leaky gut are symptoms themselves, signs that there's something going on that needs to be addressed[xiv]. And taking a random supplement isn't the answer.

Now, before we go on, we do want to highlight a key point that we just made: Your symptoms *are* real. You deserve good medical care and a doctor who will take your symptoms seriously. A doctor who is dismissive or disrespectful when you ask about leaky gut or adrenal fatigue is not doing their job correctly. You deserve to get to the bottom of what's bothering you, and you deserve to feel healthy. Too often, young women are dismissed by doctors when complaining about gut issues, period pain and inexplicable fatigue, or it's just labeled as 'stress.' This isn't right. But please, don't turn to social media for answers if this sounds familiar. You can find a practitioner who can help you. (Head to Chapter 22 for exactly how to do this.)

But back to leaky gut and adrenal fatigue 'cures.' There aren't any simple ones. That's all there is to it. No single supplement or protocol will magically heal you. It's going to be a process.

With regards to the ever-popular-on-social-media adrenal fatigue, while you absolutely could have a dysfunction with your adrenal glands, the symptoms often associated with it are the exact same as the symptoms present with low energy availability and REDs: Persistent fatigue, loss of appetite, weakness, muscle aches, feeling not energized, being unable to focus or concentrate.

Leaky gut is similar: the technical name is actually Intestinal Permeability, which is a real thing[xv,xvi]. It happens when those tight junctions of the gut wall are loosened up, which then allows more to get in, including stuff we don't want in our gut. We often see intestinal permeability with a lot of inflammation and stress. Overtrained athletes can experience it because they're training too much and not eating enough to support optimal function.

And it's a vicious cycle: not eating enough is also going to impact our gut, and then we start to assume it's because we can't tolerate things like gluten or dairy, so we restrict more and more, eat less and less, and harm our gut even more in the process.

If this sounds like you, start by stepping back and looking at the basics: Are you eating enough nutrient-dense food consistently throughout the day, managing your stress and getting enough sleep? If you're not doing those things, no supplement or test is going to help. And if you do believe that you have gut or adrenal/thyroid issues, talk to your doctor! (We know we sound like a broken record.

But the reality is that most of these deeper issues require medical intervention!)

ANY IV ANYTHING

First of all, if you're competing in the NCAA, USports, or any sport subject to anti-doping rules based on WADA[xvii] (e.g., CCES or USADA), IVs of any type are generally forbidden outside of emergency room or therapeutic use exemption (TUE) situations that have been okayed by a doctor[xviii]. Period, full stop.

But these days, influencers and wellness guru-types are popping up in your feed showing IV drips snaking into their veins as they get infusions of NAD, B vitamins, or even just pure saline hydration. Medspas (medical spas) are advertising IV drips, and even at some major marathons and other endurance sport events, IV drips are being showcased in expo areas. Unless it's done through your doctor to address a need and—if needed—you've filed the appropriate TUE, IVs are just not a good idea for young athletes. Unauthorized IV drips are unnecessary, potentially unsafe, definitely expensive, and absolutely not worth risking your athletic career over. End of story.

ANYTHING TO PREVENT/TREAT INFLAMMATION

Inflammation gets a bad rap. We hear about it as this bad thing that's making us slow and puffy, or hear that it's a sign of something going awry in the body. But inflammation is the body's natural response to injury or infection—it's your natural defense mechanism[xix]. It kickstarts your body's rebounding from training, since training causes tiny microtears in your muscles[xx]. It helps your body heal[xxi], which is the exact thing you need to do after a hard training session! This is how we get faster and stronger.

If you're sick or injured, your body is in inflammation overdrive as it works to heal. But we also see this after workouts and hard sessions. When you're fueling and sleeping enough, and not training too much, the inflammation that's happening is usually positive and the correct amount. When your body has the right resources, it's going to be able to respond to that inflammation and use that information to repair and recover your muscles, bringing down the inflammation naturally.

Yes, inflammation can be a problem when you're not giving your body the sleep or the resources it needs to recover from those training sessions, or when you're going too hard in training all the time. In those cases, you aren't giving your body the space to recover between sessions and letting those inflammation levels decrease. That's when we see chronic, elevated inflammation, and that's when it can have negative impacts, not just on performance, but overall health.

However, no supplement is going to solve inflammation—like almost every other issue, for athletes, inflammation can be solved by fueling and hydrating enough, not overdoing training, and getting enough rest and recovery. There are medical times when inflammation is an issue (see: every episode of *House, MD*) but in those cases, a supplement recommended by a social media influencer isn't the solution, a visit to your doctor is in order.

PUTTING IT ALL TOGETHER

You've read the book, *and you understand that you have to fuel. But you're a busy student-athlete, so how do you make it all actually work? In this section, we're pulling it all together so that no matter what your schedule or lifestyle looks like, you can make time for solid nutrition.*

16 / EATING AT HOME

IF YOU'RE STILL LIVING at home in high school or college, you have a great chance to learn to cook for yourself and prepare your own food in a much less stressful condition than when you're in your first apartment. Some young athletes love the idea of learning to cook (or maybe have already been cooking for themselves and their siblings for years, and if that's the case, we salute you!). But many simply rely on mom or dad to make dinner, and the extent of their cooking skill is pouring just the right amount of milk onto their cereal.

Now that you've read the rest of this book and have a better sense of what a meal should consist of and what kind of snacks and foods to eat in and around your training look like, it's time to put that into practice and actually start making these meals at home.

First, you may need to have some conversations with your parent/caregiver about what food is at home in the cupboards and fridge. Do you have what you need to make a good meal? Do you have enough easy snacks that you can grab when you're in a rush? Or are you low on carbohydrates at mealtime because your parent is on the keto diet and therefore, everyone in your family is currently stuck in low-carb land? Do your siblings snag all the bagels so you're left rummaging for snack options?

If you see that there are things missing that would help you perform at your best, like extra servings of rice with dinner and bagels in the fridge so they're easy to grab in the morning, ask to go grocery shopping with your parent, or at least ask to add a few things to the list. (We have a starter grocery list in Chapter 20 that you can share with a parent to make it even easier!)

If you have siblings who also tend to get into the snack stocks in the pantry, you may also want to ask for some shelf-stable snacks that you can hoard in your room, like trail mix or single-serve pretzels or crackers. Think about what would make it as easy as possible for you to get the food you need, when you need it.

While you're living at home, this is a great time to learn to cook a few basic meals—head to Chapter 21 for a few of our favorite easy recipes. Don't overcomplicate it. You don't need to learn to make a five course dinner or anything fancy! Maybe you could take over dinner duty one night a week, or at minimum, use this time to learn to cook the basics: Do you know how to scramble eggs, make rice, put together a tasty and filling salad, and cook an entire meal or two from scratch? You don't need to be Martha Stewart, you just need to be able to make a few things for yourself. Learn a few easy meal recipes like quesadillas, rice bowls, simple pasta dishes, stir fries, yogurt parfaits, omelets—these are all super easy to make and don't require a lot of fancy ingredients or cooking implements.

17 / EATING AT SCHOOL

EATING at school can be tricky: You start the day ultra-early as a student, and even earlier if you're in a sport that has morning practices. Your lunch may be at 10AM, but after-school practice isn't until 3PM. And the school lunches that the cafeteria offers are a joke, as are the vending machines—but who has time to pack a lunch plus all their snacks? In the last chapter, we talked about how to eat at home and talk to your parents about stocking the pantry, and hopefully we encouraged you to take a bit of ownership over the food you do bring to school... But actually making it through that school day? That's where it gets tricky.

If you have a hectic high school schedule packed with two-a-day practices, other school extracurriculars, advanced placement classes, the occasional afterschool job, et cetera, it can be really hard to eat enough throughout the day because you're just always on the move.

Start to take ownership of mealtimes by writing out your weekly schedule, including your practices, work, and class-by-class school schedule. Then, add in meal planning. What will you eat, and when will you eat it so you're fully fueled? While you don't need to follow your plan to the letter, it can be helpful to do this so you have a chart of the best times to eat, what you want to eat and drink, and what you'll need to travel with to make it happen. (See some of the sample "days in the life" in Chapter 23 for some ideas!)

When you think about your school day and your fueling, here's the simplest breakdown:

BEFORE SCHOOL

Ahh, super early mornings. It's tempting to skip breakfast in favor of hitting the snooze button a couple of extra times, but skipping your breakfast can set you back for the rest of the day—and it's hard to come back from that to be an effective student/athlete/friend/human later, especially if you pair skipping breakfast with a morning practice.

Your breakfast should be a blend of carbohydrates and protein with a bit of fat to set you up for the day, and to help you avoid the energy crash by third period. This is why it's important to establish a simple morning routine that you're going to stick to, whether that means getting to school a bit early to eat breakfast there if you can buy a bagel and a yogurt in the school cafeteria, or having your easy-to-prep smoothie ingredients ready to blend so you can drink it on the way to school, or getting up a few minutes early to make that breakfast burrito or yogurt parfait and actually taking a few minutes to just sit and eat at home. Even a glass of chocolate milk that you drink while you quickly check over your homework is a great option!

The key is coming up with a plan that is going to work for you and your schedule—and sticking to it.

AT SCHOOL

For lunch, we like to keep it simple with sandwiches. That said, having a peanut butter and jelly or turkey and provolone sandwich is a great start, but that's not enough carbohydrate for an athlete. So, add a side carbohydrate like pretzels or crackers or even some juice. Then, add some color with fruits or vegetables. If you have a heavy training session later, add an extra simple carbohydrate on top of that, like some fruit snacks or a pudding pack. A peanut butter and jelly sandwich with a piece of fruit, string cheese, a hard boiled egg and a cookie is a perfect athlete lunch. A ham and cheese sandwich with some crackers, veggies and hummus on the side is another great option.

School cafeteria food tends to be heavy on fried foods, like chicken tenders and french fries. While tasty, unfortunately these likely won't sit great in your stomach. If you are buying your lunch at school and sandwiches aren't an option, look for things that aren't deep fried. A hot pretzel with a side salad and two hard boiled eggs could be an easy option for a solid performance plate. A slice (or two) of pizza with a side salad is also great.

When lunch is at 10 AM and practice isn't until 3:30 PM, that's a long time from meal to practice, and that means you're going to need to snack in addition to eating a full lunch.

Ideally, in that situation you'll have lunch as usual in the morning, but then, you'll be able to also have a substantial snack at around 1:30 PM—another peanut butter and jelly sandwich or a soft pretzel with a string cheese is an easy option, or have something simple like yogurt and granola or a smoothie. Then, have yet another small snack like a granola bar or applesauce pouch an hour before practice if possible.

Always have easy options on hand. That means keeping emergency snacks in your locker. Things like trail mix, applesauce pouches, single-serve gummy bears, pretzels, granola bars or crackers, and a spare water bottle can be extremely helpful for the days where you forgot to bring lunch, didn't have time for a more elaborate snack, or are just feeling hungrier than usual.

Depending on your teachers and your schedule, you may be able to eat these meals and snacks in class or study hall, but if teachers have strict 'no eating' policies, you may need to snack as you walk from class to class. It can be helpful to have some of your meals and snacks be liquid in those cases—it's hard for a teacher to tell a student they can't drink a smoothie or drink a carton of chocolate milk in study hall! If you do feel like your teachers are making it hard for you to eat enough so you feel fueled at practice, though, talk to your coach about it. They can often help advocate for you so that teachers give you the green light to eat during class.

Finally, always be sipping—it can be hard to stay hydrated in high school if you don't carry a water bottle with you at all times. Even though it's a pain to carry, the bigger the water bottle, the easier it is to meet your hydration goals. And we promise you'll feel more awake and alert throughout the day!

DURING PRACTICE

Head back to Chapter 8 about how to fuel your training for the specifics, but you should never be at a practice empty-handed. Have a water bottle with some sports drink or plain water with some easy to digest carbohydrates like fruit snacks in your gym bag.

AFTER PRACTICE

If you're heading right home to dinner after practice, that meal can serve as your post-workout recovery meal. Still, you should have some water to sip on and a small snack that contains carbs and protein. If it'll be a while before you eat dinner, your post-workout snack should be much more substantial, like another sandwich or wrap.

18 / EATING IN THE DORM

COLLEGE FRESHMEN typically are required (or at least, heavily recommended) to live in the dorms at school. And that means eating at the dining hall or trying to keep your dorm room from being overrun by ants as you cook meals on a tiny hot plate or in the microwave. If you're not using a dining hall pass, skip this chapter and head to the next one about eating in your first apartment, but if you're hitting the dining hall or getting takeout for most meals and only stashing the most basic snacks in your dorm room, read on.

The key is simplicity when it comes to dealing with the dining hall. Think about building a performance plate, but don't overthink it. Focus on leaving the dining hall feeling full, satisfied and ready to crush practice rather than stressing about every single food decision, like whether or not you should hit the soft-serve machine for dessert. (The answer is almost always yes—there will be no other time in your life where you have easy access to free soft-serve ice cream.)

The dining hall can be tricky to navigate when you're first starting out at school. You're hungry, you're a little overwhelmed, and frankly, you're pretty stoked that you finally have dominion over your meal time. It makes perfect sense that you'd go a little wild at first with the more fast food-y options available, especially if your household growing up was pretty anti-fast food. Fried chicken, french fries and soda for dinner? Why not! Pancakes, bacon and a whipped mochachino for breakfast? Sure! Chicken nuggets and onion rings for lunch? Of course!

But while admittedly delicious, these heavy meals are high in fat, low in nutrient-dense foods, lacking fruits and vegetables and therefore fiber and other key micronutrients, and are generally going to sit heavy in your gut when you do head to practice. Yes, as an athlete, you do need to eat a lot, and that means there is room for some of these heavier, highly-processed foods as part of a healthy diet. But every meal shouldn't begin and end with something that's been deep fried.

The caveat here: We don't mean skip fried chicken all the time. We're talking about *balancing* your plate. If you have a piece of fried chicken, pair it with some grilled or steamed vegetables or hit the salad bar for a side salad with some dark leafy greens. Add some rice instead of french fries to get your carbohydrates, and start with water as your beverage of choice.

When building your plate, think protein, carbohydrate, and fiber (in the form of a fruit or vegetable). For example, grilled chicken breast, rice and stir fried vegetables is a perfect example of a simple meal option. Put that into a wrap or onto a sandwich and you have an easy lunch!

Get to know where things live in the dining hall and plan accordingly. In the morning, don't do a lap to decide what's for breakfast, head straight to the cereal station or the omelette bar. Knowing what you'll have in advance makes it easier to make good decisions.

It may be helpful to think about the 80:20 rule here, when it comes to balancing *healthy* and *fun*: Try to make 80 percent of your plate as nutrient-dense as possible, and leave yourself 20 percent of your plate or tray for fun. Skip the concept of 'cheat meals' or 'cheat days' entirely and instead just try to make every meal include at least one serving of fruits or vegetables and a protein plus whatever treat you're craving, and that will go a long way towards helping you stay on track to fuel your training and the rest of your life without letting food anxiety take over. And if a meal opens with fried chicken and ends with ice cream, no judgment whatsoever. The fittest, fastest athletes we know allow themselves to indulge guilt-free!

Some great 80:20 combinations could include:

- A salad topped with grilled chicken and a side of sweet potato fries
- Orange chicken, but with a lot of steamed vegetables and brown rice as your base
- Blueberry pancakes with a side of scrambled eggs and coffee with skim milk
- A burrito bowl, but with double protein and vegetables, a scoop of guacamole and a lot of fresh salsa
- Pizza with meat and veggie toppings plus a side salad

Ultimately, we don't want you to start freaking out about eating too many treats at the dining hall. You're a young athlete, you need the energy. Simply being aware of what a performance plate should look like will go a long way towards helping with your decision process.

Once you know what's served at the dining hall (most have menus available online and tend to stick to fairly regular rhythms from day to day), you can start to plan your meals a bit. Having go-to breakfasts, lunches and dinners doesn't make you boring, it just helps you streamline the process. If you never walk over to the fried chicken station, you never have to do the internal debate over whether the extra crispy is worth it. If the fried chicken is the highlight of your week, though, then you know that on Thursday, you fill your plate with salad and rice and top it with those two pieces of chicken.

It's totally okay if you deviate from your meal plans, and you absolutely should if you're feeling particularly hungry or in the mood for something different. But it's easier to start from a routine set of meals than it is to reinvent what you're eating every day—you don't have time for that!

TAKE IT TO GO

You didn't hear it from us, but getting a couple plastic or glass containers to grab a few snacks while you're in the dining hall is a great way to make sure you're snacking throughout the day. Stash some extra cereal, make a sandwich, or simply put your leftovers into a small container to eat later. Use this opportunity to fill water bottles with both water and fruit juice if you're heading to practice and need some free sports drink options or fill one with chocolate milk if you're looking for a post-workout recovery snack. Apples, bananas, trail mix and cookies are also easy ways to ensure that you have a steady stream of fuel coming in during training—and they're almost always readily available at the dining hall.

19 / EATING IN YOUR FIRST APARTMENT

WHEN YOU FIRST move away from home, it can be a little scary. Many college freshmen take advantage of living in the dorms and eating at the dining hall to bridge the gap between those home-cooked meals and grocery trips that you didn't need to make. But stepping into the real world where the pantry doesn't magically restock hurts a little bit. It takes some getting used to, but we promise you *can* feed yourself, and feed yourself well!

In this section, we're helping get your kitchen stocked, teaching you to meal plan and prep for the week ahead, helping you shop for groceries even on a tight budget, navigating a strategy for enjoying takeout, and sharing a few simple yet tasty recipes that anyone can master.

STOCK YOUR KITCHEN

Before you can start cooking your own meals, you're going to need to stock your kitchen with some basic cooking accessories. A word to the wise: Don't overdo it when you first build out your kitchen. We know you're tempted by that air fryer! But stick to the basics and add gadgets sparingly.

If you're on a tight budget, head to nearby thrift stores. You can always find things like plates and bowls there for next to nothing, and often can find things like skillets, blenders and a lot of the other stuff on this list.

- For one person, aim to have at least two plates, bowls, mugs, glasses, forks, spoons, knives, etc.
- Good chef's knife
- Cutting board
- Microwave
- Skillet with lid
- Spatula
- Single serve blender
- Medium-sized saucepan with lid
- Baking sheet
- Toaster oven or toaster
- Mixing bowl
- A couple of glass or plastic storage containers for leftovers/meal prepping
- Dishwashing equipment: Dishwasher tabs if you have a dishwasher, a sponge or scouring cloth or brush, dish soap and a couple of dishtowels will get you started
- Nice to have: Rice cooker, slow cooker or pressure cooker

Once you've built out your kitchen setup, you can start meal planning and grocery shopping.

MEAL PREP TIPS

Meal prepping starts in a notebook, not on the cutting board. While social media may make you think that meal prepping is a glamorous weekend activity involving looking somewhat stylish in your kitchen with a lot of mason jars (why is it *always* mason jars?), meal prep actually starts with looking in your cabinets and fridge to see what you already have, writing out your meal plans for the week, making a grocery list based on that, going to the grocery store to get what's on the list, unpacking that into your fridge and cabinets, and then finally getting to the cool social media-y part where you're actually meal prepping.

Think about each piece of the meal as you plan your prep, especially at first. Don't write 'salad with chicken,' list the vegetables you want to add, the rice (or other carb) that will go on top, the chicken, and the dressing you want to use. Otherwise, you'll likely forget the dressing at the store when you do get to the grocery shopping step!

Also think about portion size both pre-grocery shop and during your meal prep. Do you have enough rice for four nights? That's about two cups of rice to prep. Chicken for two nights? You'll need about a pound. Make sure you buy enough *and* that you prep enough. You'll have some missteps at first as you figure out how much you actually eat at mealtimes. You may end up with some leftovers that go uneaten, or days when you have to add a piece of toast with peanut butter after dinner because you ran out of rice. It's all a learning experience and you'll slowly get better at it!

Finally, as you plan out the food you need for the week, don't sleep on your snacks! Make sure you're adding them into your meal prep list if needed. Things like simple breads and muffins are easy to bring along to practice and can be baking in the oven as you do the rest of your meal prep for the week.

This all may sound like a lot, and if it does—and you have no idea what recipes to make—you can even use ChatGPT to help you come up with a meal plan for the week based on what you already have in your pantry, while also creating a grocery list on a budget for the items you will need. It won't be perfect, but it is a good starting point if you're feeling completely overwhelmed. (See Chapter 24 for the prompt we used and the response it gave us!)

Finally, be boring. Your meal prep doesn't need to take hours or look like a Pinterest image. The simpler you can keep each piece of prep, the better. Forget pre-making a risotto or perfectly roasting a chicken. Think "minimum viable cooking option."

As you plan out your meals for the week, think about what you can prep ahead of time that will make each meal easier. Can you....

- Pre-cook and shred chicken for salads and sandwiches
- Season and cook ground beef into crumbles for easy burrito bowls
- Clean and chop raw veggies and fruit for easy snacks and salads
- Hard boil eggs for quick breakfasts/snacks
- Measure the dry ingredients for yogurt parfaits and/or overnight oats in single-serve containers
- Cook several servings of rice or pasta (for cold pasta salad, not for hot pasta dishes!)
- Mix/pre-portion snacks like trail mix
- Bake any breads, cookies or muffins for easy carbohydrates

This will help create your to-do list for the meal prep you'll do after you grocery shop.

Get used to making time for meal prep. Make sure it (and grocery shopping) are actually written out on your schedule for the week, otherwise you'll be trying to cram them in when you're already out of food, rather than when you actually have the time.

Completely new to cooking? Don't try recipes from a Martha Stewart cookbook. Master making overnight oats, then move onto hard-boiled eggs. Start with buying pre-cooked chicken for your salads and bowls at first, then graduate to cooking your own. Learn the basics of cooking, one skill at a time. It can easily get super messy and incredibly overwhelming if you go from no cooking at all to dozens of ingredients spread on the counter waiting to be prepped.

. . .

MEAL PREP WORKSHEET

Create your own or copy this meal prep worksheet (or download the PDF version from StrongGirlPublishing.com/power-up)! We've included two versions of meal prep, one for athletes with schedules that vary from day to day enough that you won't have a "normal" eating schedule most days, and one that assumes Monday to Friday look fairly similar in terms of daily eating. Once you plan for the week, use the next worksheet to make your grocery list for the week!

WEEKLY MEAL PLANNER

	MEALS (INC. SNACKS)	INGREDIENTS
MONDAY		
TUESDAY		
WEDNESDAY		
THURSDAY		
FRIDAY		
SATURDAY		
SUNDAY		

WEEKLY MEAL PLANNER (SIMPLE)

WEEKDAY	INGREDIENTS
BREAKFAST	
LUNCH	
SNACKS	
DINNERS	

SATURDAY		

SUNDAY		

Then, use this to create your shopping list:

WEEKLY MEAL PLANNER

WHAT I HAVE ALREADY	NEED AT THE GROCERY STORE

GROCERIES ON A BUDGET

We want to be realistic and talk about money here—we know that many student athletes don't have a ton of cash on hand, and that means you're hitting the grocery store with a limited budget. So, how can you get the most nutrition for your buck?

Meal plan. There's a reason we started with that section! Meal planning helps you avoid buying random extras that will just end up going bad in the fridge.

Keep it simple. On the note of meal planning, we said it before and we'll say it again: Be boring. Have the same breakfast, lunch and snacks every day, and the same rotation of a few dinners throughout the week. This keeps your grocery list short and avoids random spice/sauce purchases that will only be used once.

Look at your grocery list from your last trip. Are there any big spends that stand out? Things like sparkling water can add up and make your trip much pricier. For the items you're splurging on, consider if there's a lower-cost (or one-time cost) alternative. Can you get a SodaStream instead of buying two cases of LaCroix every week? Or, if pricey smoothies are your thing, can you make them at home with a blender you buy secondhand?

Bulk buy. It's always cheaper to buy the big bag of rice rather than the single serve premade packets. It is an extra step, since cooking the rice rather than microwaving it takes more time, but it can save you a significant amount of money each month. (The only bulk buy we wouldn't recommend is dried beans, because they are *a lot* of work to soak and cook. Look for canned beans on sale instead!)

Shop seasonally for fresh fruits and veggies—look at what's cheaper than usual, because that's a good sign it's in season.

Don't sleep on generic store brands. Fig Newtons are a great pre- and in-workout snack, but they're pricey compared to the store brand! Ditto any kinds of crackers, cookies, cereals, and even frozen/canned fruits and veggies. Just do a quick comparison of ingredient lists to make sure they're actually similar.

Frozen veggies and fruit (especially when on sale) are a great cheaper alternative to fresh, and in some ways, we actually prefer them for student athletes, since they won't go bad if you have a busy week and opt for takeout a couple extra times. They're also easier to add to takeout meals to get some bonus veggies in there—a serving of frozen broccoli or spinach takes two minutes to microwave and is easy to eat in a few bites.

Stick to a once-a-week grocery shopping schedule whenever possible. Grocery budgets start to get out of control if you go to the store several times a week—instead, go once and only go back if you miscalculated drastically and truly need something. Otherwise, if you run low on food during the week, use it as a time to get creative with what you do have in the pantry!

Have a few 'emergency backups' that are always in the house. This could be a loaf of bread or sleeve of bagels in the freezer, a spare jar of peanut butter in the cabinet, a couple cans of your favorite soup, some granola bars—just have enough backups that if your week gets away from you, you have options in the house and don't need to resort to takeout or skipping a meal altogether because there's nothing to eat.

Prioritize your cash for foods that do matter to you. For example, while we did say buying rice in bulk is cheaper, if you know that you come home late from practice and are starving/don't have time to wait 30 minutes for rice to cook, the quick cooking single-serve rice is a smart purchase for you. Or if you're picky when it comes to the fruits and veggies you do enjoy eating, you may skip our 'seasonal produce' tip in favor of buying strawberries year-round. It's not about cutting out the foods that are convenient and your personal favorites, it's about saving money on foods that don't matter as much to you.

TAKEOUT TIPS

Let's not pretend that you won't ever order takeout. We love a good pizza night or the occasional Indian curry, and no one can deny that it sometimes feels necessary to just relax and place an order on an app rather than cooking a whole meal.

There are a few simple ways to boost the healthfulness of your order, though!

For starters, don't make takeout a regular occurrence. Weekly, or even a couple of times per week, is completely normal. But if you notice that you're opening up UberEats on the daily, it's time to work on your grocery shopping and meal prepping skills, because takeout should be a fun, occasional treat. Even if you're ordering from a salad place and the meal fits the performance plate framework perfectly, it's a bad habit to get into, and a huge money drain.

Ideally, takeout meals are planned into your week and even written out on your meal prep chart. This way, you can look forward to getting your favorite hoagie or burrito bowl or pizza, and you're doing it in a purposeful way that maximizes the enjoyment rather than in a stressed out "I don't know what to eat tonight so I'm going to have a chalupa" situation.

Make sure you're not going overboard, especially depending on the timing of your next practice. It's easy to overdo the late night ordering when you're really hungry, going for the ultra-deep-fried mozzarella stick and french fry sandwich, but if you have morning practice, your stomach is likely not going to be thrilled in the morning.

As you plan your order, break each meal into parts to see how they fit into a performance plate. For example, if you're ordering Chinese food, you can start with rice as your base carbohydrate, then add your vegetables and chicken. We're not going to tell you to skip the sauce, but if you know they tend to go heavy on the sauce, ask for it light or on the side. Steamed food is always going to be healthier than fried—but if you don't have practice in the morning and don't need to worry if the fried food sits heavy in your gut, we aren't judging an order of General Tso's chicken.

Mexican food tends to be great for healthier takeout options. You can usually build a bowl with a base of rice, add some protein, beans and vegetables, and top it with salsa and other vegetable topping—including the guacamole! If you want to maximize the health side of things, skip the heavier creamy toppings in favor of vegetable-based ones like pico de gallo, but if you love cheese, again, don't deny yourself.

Pizza is another favorite, and can even be a great pre-competition carb-loading meal. On a normal night, though, make sure you're adding a side of veggies to your takeout pizza. You can be lazy with this: A premade side salad or a microwaveable bag of frozen broccoli are easy options.

Finally, please don't stress about the occasional night out with friends or a night where you forget about the performance plate and just order exactly what you're in the mood for. The mark of a healthy, happy athlete is that you're able to go to a restaurant and order confidently, not stressing about the calories on your plate or if it's the 'perfect' performance plate. Enjoyment of food is important too!

20 / GROCERY SHOPPING 101

HERE, we're sharing a basic grocery list to get you started if you're new to shopping for yourself. You definitely don't always need everything on this list, and you should start to build one out that just features your favorites. But this can be helpful to get you started in the grocery store.

A few notes before you shop:

- Depending on your budget, you'll have to make some tricky decisions here—we've tried to keep these lists pretty simple so that you have a lot of choices and can choose less expensive options as needed. (Head back to our grocery shopping on a budget tips if you need to save cash!)
- We've listed a lot of options in each category, but you don't need to buy them all every week. For instance, you only need enough protein for seven dinners, which could consist of a pound of ground beef, a small pack of chicken, and a block of tofu. Similarly, you don't need 15

different fruits and vegetables: Choose the ones that you like and know how to prepare!
- Try to keep your fresh options that will only be good for a week to just what you actually need—your goal should be to end the week having eaten all the fresh produce in the fridge, with none of it spoiling. This will take a bit of trial and error! If you know you're bad at finishing that bagged salad before it goes brown, look for frozen vegetables and only buy fresh vegetables that have a longer shelf life, like sweet potatoes, onions and apples. Skip the lettuce, which can go limp quickly.
- Always make sure you do have enough in the pantry/freezer to get an extra day or two of meals made if you don't have time to get to the grocery store on your designated day.

CARBS:

- Bread, English Muffins, Bagels (choose 100% whole wheat/grain options when available)
- Tortillas/Wraps/Pita Bread
- Cereal
- Oatmeal
- Granola Bars (Look for brands with a short ingredient list and lower added sugar)
- Pasta
- Rice, Couscous and/or Quinoa
- Potatoes (white/red/sweet)
- Crackers/Pretzels/Fig bars
- Frozen waffles
- Treats for dessert

PROTEIN:

- Eggs
- Chicken and/or Turkey (opt for boneless and skinless or ground for the easiest prep)
- Turkey and/or chicken products (sausage, bacon)
- Lean ground beef
- Sirloin/Tenderloin
- Fish (salmon, tilapia, cod)
- Shrimp
- Tuna packets
- Lean Deli Meat
- Tofu
- Milk (regular, chocolate milk)
- Plain Greek yogurt/regular yogurt
- Cheese
- String Cheese
- Beans
- Edamame
- Lentils
- Beef or Turkey Jerky
- Protein Bars (10-15 g protein)
- Protein Powder (whey, soy, pea - look for NSF Certified for Sport or Informed Choice labels)

FRUITS + VEGGIES:

- Fresh, canned (ideally in water with no added ingredients), or frozen
- Green leafy lettuce
- Spinach
- Kale
- Bagged Salad

- Broccoli
- Asparagus
- String beans
- Bell peppers
- Brussels sprouts
- Cauliflower
- Celery
- Cucumber
- Carrots
- Mushrooms
- Onions
- Squash
- Tomato
- Zucchini
- Beets
- Cabbage
- Apple
- Banana
- Berries
- Grapefruit
- Grapes
- Kiwi
- Lemon
- Lime
- Mandarin Oranges
- Mango
- Melon
- Orange
- Peaches
- Pears
- Plums
- Dried fruits (1 tablespoon = 1 serving)
- Fruit Cups (in own juice)
- 100% Fruit Juice

CONDIMENTS/SPICES

- Spices (fresh/dried)—it can be helpful to look for blends if you're new to cooking! Chili-lime, Everyday seasoning, and Italian seasoning are good spots to start
- Vinegars (balsamic, apple)
- Salsa
- Mustard
- Barbeque Sauce
- Ketchup
- Oil-based Salad Dressings
- Hummus
- Tomato Sauce
- Honey
- Maple syrup

HEALTHY FATS

- Oils (olive, canola)
- Avocado/Guacamole
- Nuts (almonds, walnuts, pistachios, peanuts)
- Nut Butter (peanut, almond, cashew)
- Olives
- Seeds
- Ground flaxseed

21 / SIMPLE RECIPES FOR HUNGRY ATHLETES

IF YOU'RE a Martha Stewart in training, you can skip this section, but if you're someone who can manage to burn water, here are a few incredibly simple recipes to get you started on your cooking journey as a busy-but-hungry athlete. Note that a lot of these recipes make multiple servings, making them perfect for meal prepping to eat for a few days.

FRUIT AND YOGURT PARFAIT: MAKES 1 SERVING

- Ingredients: 1 cup full fat plain yogurt, 1-1.5 cups granola, berries, honey
- Directions: Scoop a ½-inch layer of yogurt into a glass jar or dish, top with a layer of berries and granola, and repeat until the container is full.
- Optional: drizzle honey on the top layer and enjoy!
- Tip: Use a container with a top if you plan to bring it on the go

MICROWAVE SCRAMBLED EGGS: 2 SERVINGS

- Ingredients: 4 eggs, ¼ cup of milk, salt to taste
- Directions: Crack eggs into a microwave safe bowl, add milk and salt and whisk. Place in the microwave and cook on high for 30 seconds. Remove bowl, beat eggs and microwave for another 30 seconds. Repeat this pattern, stirring every 30 seconds for up to 2 ½ minutes. Stop when eggs are fully cooked.

OVERNIGHT OATS: MAKES 1 SERVING

- Ingredients: ½ cup rolled oats, 1 cup of milk of choice, 2 tablespoon chia or ground flax, cinnamon and honey to taste, fruit of choice
- Directions: Combine oats, milk, chia/flax, cinnamon, and fruit in a sealable container such as a mason jar. Let sit in the fridge overnight, then add honey or other topping like peanut butter before eating. Can be eaten cold or heated up in the microwave.
- Tip: Have fun with these! Mix up your fruit, nut butter, and seeds for different flavors and nutrients!

PEANUT BUTTER AND JELLY ROLL-UPS: MAKES 1 SERVING

- Ingredients: Flour tortillas, nut butter, and jelly of choice
- Directions: Lather nut butter and jelly on the tortilla, roll up in foil and go!
- Tip: If you want to add more to this snack, slice banana and sprinkle chia seeds inside too!

EASY FRIED RICE: MAKES ABOUT 4 CUPS (2-3 SERVINGS)

- Ingredients: 3 cups cooked rice, 1-2 tablespoon oil, 1 cup frozen peas and carrots, 2 eggs, soy sauce
- Directions: Cook rice ahead of time and allow it to cool, then when you're ready to make stir fry, start by scrambling the eggs in a pan and set aside. Heat oil in the pan on medium heat, then add the peas and carrots, adding rice and eggs once veggies are slightly soft. Add soy sauce to taste and serve.
- Tip: Make it a meal by adding a protein like chicken, shrimp or tofu.

BURRITO BOWLS: MAKES 4-6 SERVINGS

- Ingredients: 2 cups uncooked rice, 1 jar of salsa, 2 cans of black beans, optional pre-cooked shredded chicken, 8 oz shredded cheese, ½ teaspoon salt, ½ teaspoon cumin, ½ teaspoon garlic powder, any other toppings you'd like– shredded lettuce, avocado, tomatoes, crushed tortilla chips, etc.
- Directions: Cook the rice with the salt in a rice cooker or on the stove. While the rice is cooking, first drain and rinse, then cook the beans with the remaining seasonings. Warm up the chicken in the microwave. Once the rice and beans are cooked, build your bowls!
- Tip: This is a good recipe to make with friends because you can adjust the portions according to your performance plate needs and add whatever toppings you'd like!

PITA PIZZAS: MAKES 6 SERVINGS

- Ingredients: 6 regular sized (not low carb!) pita bread, 1 jar of pizza sauce, 8 ounces shredded mozzarella, and your choice of toppings (shredded pre-cooked chicken, pepperoni, olives, green peppers, etc.—whatever your heart desires!)
- Directions: Preheat oven to 425 degrees Fahrenheit, coat top of pita with sauce to your desired amount, sprinkle with shredded cheese and other toppings. Place assembled pitas on a baking sheet, bake for 10 minutes until the cheese is melted. Slice and allow to cool for 2-3 minutes before eating.

ROASTED POTATOES AND VEGGIES: MAKES 4 SERVINGS

- Ingredients: 1.5 pounds potatoes, 1.5 pounds carrots both cut into 1.5-inch pieces, 3 tablespoons olive oil, salt and pepper
- Directions: Preheat oven to 400 degrees Fahrenheit. Line a baking sheet with foil or parchment paper, cut potatoes and carrots into cubes, toss them in a bowl with olive oil, salt and pepper. Transfer to the baking sheet spread out on an even layer. Bake for 50-60 minutes, check and cook until crispy.
- Tip: These are great to meal prep early in the week and have in the fridge!

QUESADILLAS: MAKES 1-2 SERVINGS

- Ingredients: 2 medium tortillas, 1 bell peppers sliced thin, 1/2 onion thinly sliced, 1/2 pound pre-cooked sliced chicken breast, 1/4 teaspoon chili powder, 1/4 teaspoon cumin, 1/4 teaspoon dried oregano, 3/4 cup shredded cheddar cheese, 3/4 cup shredded Monterey Jack cheese, sour cream for serving
- Directions: In a large skillet pan, add oil on medium heat, cook peppers and onions until soft and set on a plate. Add another tablespoon of oil to the pan and add chicken, chili powder, cumin, and oregano. Cook while stirring occasionally, about 8 minutes. Transfer to a plate and wipe the pan with a paper towel. Add a tortilla to the pan, cover half with shredded cheese then add ¼ of the pepper and onion mixture and ¼ of the chicken to the cheese side. Fold the other half over, cook for 3 minutes then flip and cook the other side for 3 minutes. Cut each in half and serve.

NOT-A-SAD-SALAD: 1 SERVING

- Ingredients: Mixed greens of choice (spinach, kale, arugula, romaine lettuce, spring mix); Veggie toppings of choice (tomatoes, onion, mushrooms, peppers, etc); Pre-cooked sliced chicken or plant based alternative; 1-2 cup starchy carb (roasted sweet potato, quinoa, brown rice, big hunks of bread on the side); Dressing (*no* low-fat dressings!)
- Directions: Chop, place in a bowl and toss to combine, enjoy!

EGG BITES: MAKES 12 EGG BITES, 4-6 SERVINGS

- *Note: This is a great meal prep recipe to make once a week, but you can also cut it in half*
- Ingredients: 12 eggs, 3 cups chopped veggies (broccoli, mushrooms, pepper), ¼ cup milk, 1 teaspoon oil, ¼ cup shredded cheese, salt and pepper to taste
- Directions: Preheat oven to 350 degrees Fahrenheit. Chop veggies and cook in a pan in oil until tender. Mix the eggs, milk, and cheese in a bowl. Spray a muffin tin with cooking spray and add the veggies evenly. Then pour the egg mixture evenly. Bake for 22-25 minutes or until set. Remove and serve or allow to cool and refrigerate for later.

PASTA SALAD: MAKES 12 SERVINGS

- *Note: This is a great meal prep recipe to make once a week, but you can also cut it in half*
- Ingredients: 16 ounce box of pasta of choice, one bottle of Italian salad dressing, 2 cucumbers chopped, 6 tomatoes chopped, 1 bunch of green onions chopped, 4 ounces grated parmesan cheese, 1 tablespoon Italian seasoning
- Directions: Bring a large pot of lightly salted water to a boil. Place pasta in the pot, cook for 8 to 12 minutes and drain. Toss pasta, Italian dressing, and vegetables in a large dish. Mix the cheese and seasoning in a small dish and gently work into the pasta salad. Chill for at least 30 minutes before serving.

PASTA BAKE: MAKES 8 SERVINGS

- Ingredients: Box of penne pasta, 1 pound ground beef, 1 chopped onion, ¾ cup mushrooms, 28 ounces jar pasta sauce, 2 cups shredded mozzarella cheese
- Directions: Bring a large pot of lightly salted water to a boil. Place pasta in the pot, cook for 8 to 12 minutes and drain. Meanwhile, cook ground beef, onion, and mushrooms in a skillet on medium heat until browned. Preheat oven to 325 degrees Fahrenheit. Combine mushrooms, sauce, shredded mozzarella cheese, pasta, and ground beef and onion mixture in a large bowl. Transfer to a greased 9x13-inch casserole dish. Bake for 20-25 minutes.

SHEET PAN FAJITAS: MAKES 4 SERVINGS

- Ingredients: Fajita seasoning, 1 large onion, 3 bell peppers, 1 pound chicken, 2 tablespoons oil, 1 lime, 8 6-inch tortillas, sour cream to taste.
- Directions: Preheat oven to 400 degrees Fahrenheit. Cut the onion and bell pepper into strips. Slice chicken into thin strips. Place the veggies and chicken on a large baking sheet or casserole dish. Drizzle with oil and sprinkle seasoning. Use hands to mix until coated. Spread evenly across the baking sheet or dish. Bake for 35-40 minutes stirring halfway through. Squeeze juice from half of the lime over the meat and vegetables once they are done cooking.
- Tip: Serve in tortillas and add sour cream top if you wish. Need a moderate to hard day plate? Serve with some rice for a carb boost.

SMOOTHIE TIPS AND TRICKS

First of all, let's be clear: smoothies aren't automatically healthy. It's easy to end up on a sugar high and then have that sugar crash from sipping a smoothie that's all ice, fruit and sweetener. (It also won't fill you up!)

To make a smoothie into a meal, make sure you've added some fat and protein. A spoonful of peanut butter and a few spoonfuls of Greek yogurt will make your smoothie much more satisfying.

Need a heftier meal? Use your smoothie like the base of an Acai bowl if you want it to be more filling: Add slices of banana, granola, nuts and seeds and eat with a spoon!

Stop overcomplicating it. Your smoothie doesn't need 700 superfoods.

With these simple smoothie recipes, simply add all of the ingredients to a blender and blend until smooth. Serve and enjoy!

ULTIMATE BASIC SMOOTHIE RECIPE: MAKES 1 SERVING

- 1 cup Greek yogurt
- 1/2 cup milk
- 1 1/2 cups of your favorite frozen fruit
- Maple syrup or honey to taste

BANANA TOFU SMOOTHIE: MAKES 1 SERVING

- 1 banana
- 1/2 cup Silken Tofu
- 3 tablespoons hemp seeds
- 1 tablespoon maple syrup
- 1/2 teaspoon cinnamon
- 1 cup soy milk

BERRY OAT SMOOTHIE: MAKES 1 SERVING

- 1 cup milk
- 1/4 cup blueberries
- 1/2 banana
- 1/3 cup strawberries
- 5 ice cubes
- 1 scoop vanilla protein powder or ¾ cup Greek yogurt
- 1/4 cup oats
- 2 teaspoons hemp seeds
- 1 tablespoon nut butter

TROPICAL SMOOTHIE: MAKES 1 SERVING

- 1/3 cup frozen pineapple
- 1/3 cup frozen mango
- 2 tablespoon frozen avocado
- 1/2 cup orange juice
- 1/2 cup milk
- 1 scoop vanilla protein powder or 3/4 cup Greek yogurt
- 1/2 cup spinach (optional)

22 / HOW TO TALK TO EXPERTS— AND BE TAKEN SERIOUSLY

We've mentioned the idea of talking to your doctor or a dietitian a bunch of times throughout this book. But it's often easier said than done. How do you show up at the office prepared with the right questions and the right information to be taken seriously? We know that often, doctors are overworked and tend to, well, gloss over or dismiss when a fit-looking young woman shows up complaining of stomach issues, fatigue, pain, headaches, hair loss, or any number of scary symptoms.

In fact, a 2019 survey[i] found that over 50 percent of women believe gender discrimination in patient care is a serious problem, while one in five women surveyed reported feeling ignored or dismissed by a healthcare provider.

That means in order to get the help you need, especially if you're using the university's medical system, you may need to show up to the doctor fully prepared and ready to advocate for yourself.

DON'T ACCEPT A NON-DIAGNOSIS (WITHOUT A PLAN)

Often, young women are given a "diagnosis of exclusion," a diagnosis that's given because other diagnosable conditions have been ruled out, like irritable bowel syndrome (IBS)[ii]. They're often told that their symptoms are "caused by stress" because it's the easiest way to say "we don't really know what's wrong but we don't want to investigate it anymore." In fact, women are twice as likely as men to receive that IBS diagnosis[iii]. And yes, that may be a legitimate and accurate diagnosis, but if it doesn't come with a management plan, it's not very helpful.

Women are also twice as likely to be diagnosed with depression or anxiety, which again, can be very real diagnoses[iv]. Unfortunately, sometimes these diagnoses can be missing a physical element that's actually contributing to those issues. And the worst is the diagnosis of "stress." Yes, it's very possible that your gut/performance/fatigue symptoms are brought on by or exacerbated by stress. But if a doctor doesn't do any testing and immediately skips to stress, that's a red flag.

If you feel as though your doctor is diagnosing you with one of these "non-diagnoses" without much testing, or without a treatment or follow-up plan, ask more questions—and if they won't budge on testing, it may be time to look for a second opinion. (We're big fans of getting second opinions.)

Be ready to advocate for yourself. The average length of a doctor's appointment is around 15 minutes[v], with roughly five minutes of it spent with the patient (that's you) actually talking. Give yourself a pep talk before you head in—no one cares more about your health than you, and you need to make the doctor care enough (or get curious enough) to help you get to the bottom of what's going on. That may mean asking a question twice, asking for clarification, asking for a referral, or asking for a specific test.

If you're not sure you'll be able to do this, it's okay to bring a parent, a trusted adult, or even a good friend with you to help you advocate for yourself.

Here are a few tips for advocating for yourself at the doctor's office:

BE PREPARED

- Show up with a symptoms list that's written out so you don't forget anything. Get specific: How high was your fever? How long has the pain been going on? What have you tried in order to solve it?
- Bring a food diary from the last week. It doesn't need to be perfect, but it can be helpful for your doctor, dietitian or therapist to see what you're eating rather than asking about it and you trying to recall what you had for breakfast on Tuesday. Dietitians also love to see photos of your food so they can get a rough idea of your regular portion sizes.
- Bring a list of any supplements you're taking, medications you've been on, or previous issues you may have had that could be related. If you've had any testing done in the last couple of years that you can access, bring that as well.
- Have a writeup of your last month's training schedule, in case the doctor or dietitian asks about training specifics. (Often, athletes are automatically assumed to be overtraining, and while that may be the case, it's not always the answer!)

DON'T BE AFRAID TO ASK FOLLOW-UPS

Ask for clarifications around diagnoses, rehab from injury, or any health related topic, including your menstrual cycle.

Don't be afraid of feeling ashamed or embarrassed of not knowing a medical term or more about how your body works—your providers are there to help educate and support you.

This could look like...

- Asking what a normal cycle should be like, including symptoms that you feel throughout especially if they feel like they are impacting your ability to complete coursework or perform in sport
- How you can use a period tracker to learn more about your symptoms and how they impact your well-being.
- Being straightforward about how you are feeling mentally —especially if you're feeling down or unusually anxious
- Asking for a clearer explanation of what an injury is and what the healing and rehab process will be for you so you can make a safe return to sport

If you ask for more information or do not feel you have your questions answered, be straightforward that you do not understand and ask for it to be explained to you in a different way.

Some great ways to do this are saying:

"Can you help me understand...?"

"When will results be available?"

"What are the next steps?"

ENLIST YOUR COACH/TRAINER/THERAPIST

Unfortunately, sometimes it's easier for a doctor to take a coach seriously compared to a young athlete. It's wrong, but sometimes, that's simply the reality. For example, if you're worried that LEA is becoming an issue or you're concerned your iron might be low based on a decrease in your performance, your coach can attest to that decrease and turn it from feeling to fact in the eyes of the doctor. If you suspect that your doctor would be more willing to assess your symptoms seriously if your coach could back you up, consider asking your coach to phone, send an email, or even write a short message for you to bring in confirming what your symptoms are. This is especially true if you're using the university healthcare system, since if you're a student-athlete, you should have access to sports medicine experts.

ASK FOR A REFERRAL

Often, doctors are busy and not overly keen on pursuing a line of testing that they'll have to deal with, especially if they aren't sure there's an issue to begin with. If you suspect your doctor isn't going to be overly helpful at figuring out what's wrong, you can ask for a referral to a specialist who might have more answers. A gynecologist or endocrinologist may be more inclined to do a full hormone panel, while a registered dietitian can help assess if you may have REDs or LEA. For injury issues, asking for a referral for physical therapy may get you in for treatment sooner. And because the healthcare system, especially in the US, can be a bit... impossible to deal with, having these referrals can help you avoid costly out-of-pocket feed and streamline the insurance process.

ASK FOR/SEEK OUT A SECOND OPINION

If you don't feel like a doctor listened to you, it's okay to go to another doctor for a second opinion. (Hot tip: You can even mention that to the doctor as they try to end the appointment. Ask for a recommendation. At minimum, this lets them know that they haven't done a very good job at helping you. It may even prompt them to order a few extra tests.)

TAKE ADVANTAGE OF FREE/LOW-COST SERVICES AND TESTING THAT YOU DO HAVE ACCESS TO

If you're a university student, you likely have access to basic medical care at the student health center—but you may have access to even more than that! Many universities offer free or low-cost access to mental health services and even dietitians, optometrists and other experts. If you're a student athlete, you likely have even greater access to sports medicine experts and will be able to access things like sweat rate testing, bloodwork, DEXA scans and more. Even if you're not a student athlete, check in at the school's fitness center, since some of the fitness centers offer things like low cost sweat testing and more. Trust us, there is no better time to do a deep dive on health than when you're in school. It will never be cheaper or easier!

Depending on where you live in the world, you may or may not have private health insurance. If you do, get to know your policy: you may be surprised what's actually covered. Some plans will cover physical therapy even without a referral, while others will cover a visit to a dietitian without a referral—though there may be a co-pay or deductible.

23 / SAMPLE DAYS IN THE LIFE

WE KNOW it can be hard to read all of that information and put it into practice as a busy athlete. It's tough to actually visualize how you'd really eat like an athlete while living in the dorm, how to pack snacks for a full day of two practices plus school, or how you would fuel while away on a weekend trip. So here, we're sharing a few sample schedules of different young women athletes and how they optimally fuel even the busiest day. No two athletes are the same, so you won't copy their food logs exactly, but it may help you plan your meals for the week and even think about your eating schedule in a new way.

Remember, these are just meant to be examples, not perfect blueprints for "the right" day of eating. You may be an athlete who needs more carbohydrates to feel her best, or requires an extra snack before bedtime. How you fuel is individual to you and will vary day by day based on your activity levels, your hormones, and so many other factors, from how well to slept to how stressed you are.

SOPHIE

Age: 20 years old
Sport: NCAA D1 Volleyball
Season: Currently in-season with daily practice and tournaments
Living: In a dorm

- 6:30 AM: Wake up, morning nutrition and hydration: banana and water bottle with electrolytes
- 7:00 AM: Light stretching and pre-breakfast mobility
- 7:30 AM: Breakfast: at a cafe on campus, bagel and egg sandwich, a black coffee, and a fruit cup
- 8:00 AM - 9:30 AM: Kinesiology 305
- 9:30 AM: Snack: applesauce pouch
- 10:00 AM - 11:30 AM: Strength and Conditioning
- 12:00 PM: Lunch: at the dining hall: stir fry with rice, veggies, and tofu and a glass of chocolate milk
- 1:00 PM - 2:30 PM: Sports Psychology 320 (Team Dynamics lecture)
- 3:00 PM - 4:30 PM: Study Date at Campus Library, snack of trail mix and an apple
- 5:30 PM - 7:30 PM: Evening Volleyball Skills Training
- 8:00 PM: Dinner: at the dining hall with teammates: pasta with chicken and a side salad, cookie
- 9:30 PM: Light stretching, foam rolling: snack on Greek yogurt and granola in dorm
- 10:30 PM: Bedtime for optimal recovery

Why it works: Sophie had carbs at all of her meals and packed snacks to munch on during her busy day! No meal was low carb, which is key for someone with two-a-day practices.

JENNIFER

Age: 15 years old
Sport: Cross-country running
Season: Currently in-season with daily practice
Living: At home

- 5:30 AM: Wake up, light stretching
- 5:45 AM: Pre-workout nutrition: Pop-Tart and water
- 6:00 AM: Morning easy training run
- 6:50 AM: Cool down, shower, and get ready for school
- 7:15 AM: Oatmeal topped with walnuts, honey, and berries
- 7:45 AM - 12:30 PM: Classes
- 10:00 AM: Snack in between classes: muffin and a string cheese
- 12:30 - 1:00 PM: Lunch from home, turkey sandwich with veggies and hummus on top, pretzels, an apple and peanut butter
- 1:00 - 3:00 PM: Classes, quick snack while getting ready: fig bars
- 3:00 - 4:30 PM: Cross-country team practice, small bottle of chocolate milk on the way home
- 5:30 PM: Dinner with family, grilled burger on a bun, side of steamed broccoli and potato wedges with ketchup, glass of apple juice
- 6:00 PM - 8:00 PM: Homework and study time, two scoops of ice cream with chocolate sauce
- 9:00 PM: Bedtime (aim for 8-9 hours of sleep)

Why it works: Jen enjoyed her favorite food— ice cream—before bed, and goes to bed early enough to get 8 hours of sleep despite the early wakeup time!

EMMA

Age: 14
Sport: High school swimmer
Season: Off-season
Living: At home

- 6:30 AM: Homemade yogurt parfait with granola and fruit, bottle of orange juice
- 7:00 AM: Pack lunch, get ready, leave for school
- 8:00 AM: Classes
- 10:00 AM: Granola bar and dried fruit
- 12:00 PM: Lunch break with friends, two slices of pizza from the cafeteria with a side salad
- 3:00 PM: Commute home
- 3:30 PM: Bowl of cereal with a banana and light stretching
- 4:00 PM: Homework/study session and a walk with a friend
- 6:00 PM: Dinner with family: chicken with roasted potatoes and veggies
- 7:00 PM: Review for upcoming tests/projects
- 8:00 PM: Watch TV, peanut butter toast with honey
- 9:00 PM: Prepare for bed (shower, pack swim gear for the next morning)

Why it works: Emma shared a meal and socialized with friends while still building a performance plate that fit her training level.

ANYA

Age: 19 years old
Sport: NCAA D3 Lacrosse
Season: In-season
Living: In an off-campus apartment

- 7:00 AM: Smoothie with frozen fruit, Greek yogurt, and peanut butter
- 8:00 AM: 1 hour lift with the team
- 9:20 AM: Bagel with cream cheese
- 9:30 AM: Class, Human Growth and Development 100
- 11:00 PM: Packed lunch, sandwich with ham and veggies, tortilla chips and guacamole on-campus while studying for test
- 12:30 PM: Class, Intro to Psychology 101
- 2:00 PM: Snack: fig bars and applesauce pouch and mobility before practice
- 3:00 PM: Lacrosse practice
- 6:30 PM: Team dinner with roommates at home, lasagna (frozen) and steamed broccoli
- 8:00 PM: Study, homework and nighttime snack, bowl of cereal with milk
- 10:30 PM: Bedtime

Why it works: Anna had a bagel and a sandwich on campus and lasagna for dinner, which helped her get plenty of carbs. And her breakfast smoothie set her up for a successful morning after training without making her late for class since she could take it with her!

MIA

Age: 13 years old
Sport: High-school basketball
Season: In-season
Living: At home

- 7:30 AM: Wake up, breakfast: freezer waffles with syrup and a side of yogurt with fruit
- 8:30 AM: Final preparations for school (pack lunch, review schedule)
- 9:00 AM: Classes
- 12:00 PM: Eat lunch and socialize with friends; pasta with meatballs and side of veggies
- 2:00 PM: Snack in history class before heading to practice; sports drinks and granola bar
- 3:00 PM: Softball practice
- 5:15 PM: Snack on the ride home from practice; chicken tenders and a small fry from the drive thru
- 5:45 PM: Homework/study session
- 6:30 PM: Dinner with family; taco night with all of the fixings
- 8:00 PM: Free time
- 9:00 PM: Prepare for bed (shower, prep for school)

Why it works: Mia used freezer food as an easy way to get a performance plate at breakfast to help her stay energized through the whole day. It doesn't have to be fancy to be a healthy performance plate!

CHLOE

Age: 18 years old
Sport: NCAA D2 Water Polo
Season: In-season
Living: Dorms

- 5:30 AM: Wake up and get ready; granola bar and sports drink
- 6:00 AM: Weight room training
- 7:00 AM: Breakfast at the dining hall; omelette with toast and fruit and yogurt
- 7:30 AM: Prep for the day, light stretching
- 8:30 AM: Lecture, Macroeconomics ECO 201
- 9:30 AM: Snack and prep for test; trail mix and cookie
- 10:30 AM: Statistics ECO 207 test
- 11:30 AM: Eat lunch, socialize with friends, catch-up on homework; chicken noodle soup with a grilled cheese sandwich
- 1:30 PM: Lecture, ENG 112
- 2:30 PM: Pre-practice snack, get to gym; protein bar and dried fruit
- 3:30 PM: Film, play review, light scrimmage at the pool; sips of sports drink
- 6:15 PM: Dinner at the dining hall with teammates; chicken quesadilla, salad, and tortilla chips
- 7:00 PM: Homework and study time
- 8:00 PM: Quality time with roommates, milkshake
- 9:30 PM: Prepare for bed and the next day

Why it works: Chloe had both a pre-lift snack and still made time for a balanced breakfast after her lift to recover and repair before afternoon practice!

SARAH

Age: 21 years old
Sport: NCAA D1 Soccer
Season: In-season
Living: Women's soccer team house

- 8:00 AM: Wake up and get ready; a few sheets of graham crackers and electrolyte drink
- 8:30 AM: Captain-led team run
- 9:45 AM: Breakfast at the dining hall with the team; yogurt, fruit, and bagel with peanut butter
- 10:30 AM: PA 606 Medical Epidemiology
- 11:45 AM: Eat lunch and prep for meeting; stir fried rice with shrimp
- 1:30 PM: Meeting with clinical advisor for applied research project
- 2:30 PM: Pre-practice snack on the way to gym (vending machine gummy bears and water)
- 3:30 PM: Practice, conditioning and drills; sips of sports drink during
- 5:15 PM: Dinner with housemates; pita pizzas and salad
- 7:00 PM: Homework and research, cookie and tea
- 8:00 PM: Relax, light stretch, unwind
- 10:00 PM: Prepare for bed and clinical rotation the next day; leftover Halloween candy before bed

Why it works: Sarah made sure to have sports drink during practice to perform well and stay hydrated, and followed it up with an early dinner.

RILEY

Age: 16 years old
Sport: High school and club softball
Season: In-season
Living: At home

- 7:00 AM: Wake up, breakfast; granola with almond milk, peanut butter and berries
- 7:30 AM: Prep for school (pack lunch, review schedule)
- 8:00 AM: Commute to school
- 8:30 AM: Classes
- 10:00 AM: Half of a peanut butter and jelly sandwich
- 12:00 PM: Lunch and socialize with friends; big bowl of pasta salad and juice
- 2:00 PM: Snack in history class before heading to practice (banana and plant-based yogurt)
- 3:00 PM: Softball practice
- 5:15 PM: Snack on the ride home from practice; chia seed pudding with fruit
- 6:00 PM: Dinner with family; black bean and sweet potato chili
- 6:30 PM: Catch and skills at the park with mom
- 7:15 PM: Homework and study
- 8:30 PM: Reading time; brownie and herbal tea
- 9:00 PM: Prepare for bed (shower, prep for school)

Why it works: Riley is still eating to support her training while choosing to follow a plant-based eating pattern—and making sure meals still contain plenty of protein!

SKYLAR

Age: 17 years old
Sport: Gymnastics
Season: In-season
Living: At home

- 5:00 AM: Wake up, breakfast; toast with jelly and Greek yogurt
- 5:30 AM: Strength and conditioning session
- 6:30 AM: Shower, get ready for school; drive thru breakfast sandwich
- 7:15 AM: Commute to school
- 7:30 AM: Homework and socialize before classes
- 8:00 AM: Classes
- 10:00 AM: Peanut butter on crackers with an apple
- 12:00 PM: Lunch—tortilla chips + guac, leftover chicken quesadilla
- 2:30 PM: Snack in class class; granola bar and gummies from the vending machine
- 3:30 PM: Commute to gym
- 3:45 PM: Practice
- 7:00 PM: Recovery drink on commute home
- 7:00 PM: Dinner; roasted potatoes, veggies, and chicken
- 8:00 PM: Homework; popcorn for a snack
- 8:30 PM: Prepare for early bedtime

Why it works: Skylar may not have been perfectly prepared, but she used vending machine snacks as an option to fuel up before practice instead of skipping a pre-practice snack. She also had an early bedtime to since she had an early morning.

BRIANNA

Age: 14 years old
Sport: Ice hockey
Season: Off-season
Living: At home

- 10:00 AM: Wake up, scrambled eggs and a bagel for breakfast
- 11:00 AM: Work on school project that's due next week, text with friends
- 12:00 PM: Stir fried veggies, rice, and chicken
- 2:30 PM: Snack; protein bar and sports drink
- 3:00 PM: Skate and Sunday pickup game with friends at the rink
- 5:15 PM: Snack on the ride home; peanut butter filled pretzels and apple
- 5:45 PM: Dinner with family; crockpot beef stew with potatoes, carrots, and celery
- 6:30 PM: Homework and study
- 8:00 PM: Free time (relaxation, hobbies, or stretching) snack; chocolate peanut butter cups
- 9:00 PM: Prepare for bed (shower, prep for school tomorrow)

Why it works: Brianna slept in on the weekend to catch up on sleep, and is enjoying the offseason, but still having fun getting some movement in!

24 / USING CHATGPT AS A MEAL PLANNING TOOL

AI IS NOT A REGISTERED DIETITIAN, and shouldn't be advising you on how to eat! (Much like the human body, "garbage in, garbage out" really applies to AI learning models.) But what it can do is help you do things like meal plan and create a grocery list for the week. It won't always be perfectly accurate—but if you're new to grocery shopping and cooking on your own, it can make the task of getting ready for a week of meals ahead feel a lot less daunting.

We like using a prompt like the one below to create a meal plan, provide some basic recipe instructions, and build a grocery list, but you should tweak it to work for what you need!

Our Prompt: Create a meal plan with easy recipes that a college student athlete with minimal cooking experience could follow for a week of eating including breakfast, lunch, dinner and two snacks every day. Ideally, it will use the ingredients already in their fridge and pantry: brown rice, a can of black beans, carrots, one onion, a can of tomatoes, a half loaf of bread, some frozen spinach, olive oil, and a few apples. Also create a grocery list for the ingredients that they will still need to buy.

. . .

ChatGPT's Response:

7-DAY MEAL PLAN (INCLUDES BREAKFAST, LUNCH, DINNER, 2 SNACKS)

Day 1

- **Breakfast:** Scrambled eggs with spinach + toast
- **Snack 1:** Apple with peanut butter
- **Lunch:** Rice bowl with black beans, sautéed carrots and onions
- **Snack 2:** Greek yogurt with granola
- **Dinner:** Pasta with canned tomatoes, spinach, onion and olive oil

Day 2

- **Breakfast:** Overnight oats with chopped apple and cinnamon
- **Snack 1:** Hard-boiled egg + carrot sticks
- **Lunch:** Tuna sandwich on toasted bread + side carrots
- **Snack 2:** Trail mix (nuts + dried fruit)
- **Dinner:** Stir-fried rice with black beans, onion, carrots, spinach

Day 3

- **Breakfast:** Toast with scrambled eggs and sautéed spinach
- **Snack 1:** Apple + cheese stick
- **Lunch:** Tomato soup with rice + toast
- **Snack 2:** Hummus with carrot sticks
- **Dinner:** Chicken and veggie stir fry over brown rice

Day 4

- **Breakfast:** Greek yogurt + apple slices + oats
- **Snack 1:** Boiled egg + toast
- **Lunch:** Rice bowl with black beans, avocado, salsa, onion
- **Snack 2:** Cottage cheese + fruit
- **Dinner:** Baked potato topped with beans, spinach, and cheese

Day 5

- **Breakfast:** Oatmeal with chopped apple and cinnamon
- **Snack 1:** Banana + peanut butter
- **Lunch:** Grilled cheese + tomato soup
- **Snack 2:** Crackers + hummus
- **Dinner:** Tuna rice salad with carrots, onion, spinach

Day 6

- **Breakfast:** Toast + eggs + sautéed spinach
- **Snack 1:** Apple + granola bar
- **Lunch:** Bean and veggie wrap (use tortillas)
- **Snack 2:** Yogurt + frozen berries
- **Dinner:** Pasta with tomato-spinach sauce + cheese

Day 7

- **Breakfast:** Overnight oats with apple and nut butter
- **Snack 1:** Cheese + carrots
- **Lunch:** Brown rice with black beans, frozen corn, salsa
- **Snack 2:** Trail mix
- **Dinner:** Egg and veggie scramble with toast

Grocery List

Protein

- Eggs (1 dozen)
- Greek yogurt (plain or flavored)
- Tuna (canned, 2–3 cans)
- Cheese sticks or block cheese
- Cottage cheese
- Chicken breast (1–2 pounds or precooked)
- Hummus
- Peanut butter

Produce

- Bananas (3–4)
- Avocados (2)
- Potatoes (2–3)
- Frozen berries (1 bag)
- Frozen corn (1 bag)
- Lettuce or mixed greens (optional for wraps/bowls)

Grains and Pantry

- Rolled oats
- Pasta (1 box)
- Granola
- Granola bars (snack size)
- Whole grain tortillas or wraps
- Crackers

Extras

- Cinnamon
- Salsa

As you can see, it's not perfect. For one thing, it's definitely a bit light on the amount of food you'd need to buy (who only eats two avocados in a week, what the heck is tomato-spinach sauce, and where is the trail mix on the shopping list?)—but it's a great starting point for a new chef! It can also be helpful getting all those random things that have been in your cabinets for a while used up: Just feed them into the prompt and ask for recipes that would let you finish them up.

25 / DAILY FOOD JOURNAL TEMPLATE

Copy this journal and use it to keep track of your energy levels throughout the day—after a couple of weeks, look back at past entries to see what trends you can spot. What's working? What's not?

Day of the week: M | T | W | Th | F | S | S

Do you have your period: Y | N

Any illness/injury issues? _____

Training/competition: _____

How did you feel during? How was your energy, performance, etc.?

School/extracurriculars: How busy was your day? Did you feel like you were able to pay attention in class?

Sleep: Trouble falling asleep? Staying asleep? Waking up?

MEALS:

Breakfast:_____

Snack:_____

Lunch:_____

Snack:_____

Dinner: _____

Snack:_____

Overall Energy Rating (1-10): ____

Download the free PDF version of this log at:
StrongGirlPublishing.com/power-up

ACKNOWLEDGEMENTS

I've always been a believer of sitting at the table with people who are 'smarter' than you are—those who show up in a thoughtful yet big way. Whether it's through their consistent but quiet actions, their willingness to try and fail, or those who will never hesitate to push you because they believe you are capable. In every 'season' of life, I feel lucky to have individuals who I sit with, and without them, I certainly would not be writing the acknowledgments for my first book.

Sport has been a pillar for me for as long as I can remember, and I am forever grateful for everything it has given me. From self-confidence, an outlet on bad days, lifelong friendships, to a space where I can be my most authentic self. So thank you to my mom, Lisa, for allowing me to try ALL of the sports. I'll never forget you standing on the sidelines of every single lacrosse or soccer game–rain, snow, or shine–to standing in knee-deep water watching me race another Ironman.

A massive thank you to Molly with Strong Girl Publishing– the brains behind this book concept, my co-author, and publisher. I quite literally would not have been able to do this without you. The space you've created for us to collaborate to help support young female athletes to not only get into sport, but to stay and thrive is incredible.

For the peers who helped us bring this baby to print–Sasha, Natalie, Brooke, and Holley. I cannot thank you enough for taking your precious time and expertise to provide thoughtful feedback.

There is no better feeling than being in a field where we know collaboration will lift us all up.

And to Emma, Sarah, and the countless other friends, family, and coaches who have always been there hyping me up—you are the realest.

To the young women reading this book, I hope this sparks a shift in how you think about food and your body, not only for sport but to be able to step into your most vibrant and true self. We aren't here to make ourselves smaller, but to take up space and show the world what we're capable of.

-Stevie Lyn Smith

ABOUT THE AUTHORS

STEVIE LYN SMITH, RD

Stevie Lyn Smith is a registered dietitian and founder of Stevie Lyn Nutrition, a virtual sports nutrition private practice. Her mission is to help educate and coach athletes and active humans on how to fuel their goals while not sacrificing their health and happiness.

As a board certified specialist in sports nutrition, Stevie Lyn has helped hundreds of athletes and active individuals fuel to improve their performance, energy levels, and recovery without feelings of guilt or restriction. Drawing from her experiences growing up as a team-sport athlete to completing ten full Ironman distance triathlons and countless other endurance and ultra distance races, she knows firsthand how important nutrition is to be a healthy athlete.

She received her B.S. in Dietetics and Nutrition from SUNY Buffalo State University in 2012 and M.S. in Applied Nutrition with a Sports and Fitness concentration from Northeastern University in 2019. She is the host of her podcast, Real Fuel with SLS, where she has honest conversations to dive into the human side of endurance sports paired with sports nutrition knowledge for the everyday athlete. She has also contributed to *Run Tri Bike Magazine, Runner's World Magazine, Outside Magazine, Bicycling Magazine,* and *Triathlete Magazine.* In her free time, she enjoys volunteering at her local animal shelter. When she's not swimming, biking, or running you can find her outside exploring new trails or with her dog in sunny Buffalo, NY.

MOLLY HURFORD

Molly Hurford is the founder of Strong Girl Publishing and has been called a chronic book writer by her friends. She's a journalist by trade, and writes and speaks about all things cycling, running, nutrition and movement-related. She's the author of multiple books including *Running as Fast as We Can* and *Fuel Your Ride* as well as the Shred Girls series. She's also the co-author of *Sprinting Through Setbacks* with Micha Powell.

When not actually outside, she's probably writing about being outside or healthy habits of cyclists and runners, and interviewing world-class athletes and scientists for The Consummate Athlete podcast and website.

Molly is a little obsessed with getting people—especially girls—psyched on adventure and being outside. Those passions combined are what prompted her to start Strong Girl Publishing in order to reach more young girls and help them find and stay in sports and outdoor adventuring.

REFERENCES

INTRODUCTION

i. Sawyer, Susan M et al. "The age of adolescence." *The Lancet. Child & adolescent health* vol. 2,3 (2018): 223-228. doi:10.1016/S2352-4642(18)30022-1

ii. Brown, Kelly A et al. "Participation in sports in relation to adolescent growth and development." *Translational pediatrics* vol. 6,3 (2017): 150-159. doi:10.21037/tp.2017.04.03

1. MACRONUTRIENTS: WHAT ARE THEY + WHY DO THEY MATTER?

i. Kerksick, C.M., Wilborn, C.D., Roberts, M.D. et al. ISSN exercise & sports nutrition review update: research & recommendations. *J Int Soc Sports Nutr* 15, 38 (2018). https://doi.org/10.1186/s12970-018-0242-y

2. CARBS ARE QUEEN

i. Utter, Alan C et al. "Carbohydrate attenuates perceived exertion during intermittent exercise and recovery." *Medicine and science in sports and exercise* vol. 39,5 (2007): 880-5. doi:10.1249/mss.0b013e31803174a8

ii. Ackerman, Kathryn E et al. "Low energy availability surrogates correlate with health and performance consequences of Relative Energy Deficiency in Sport." *British journal of sports medicine* vol. 53,10 (2019): 628-633. doi:10.1136/bjsports-2017-098958

iii. Kerksick, C.M., Arent, S., Schoenfeld, B.J. et al. International society of sports nutrition position stand: nutrient timing. *J Int Soc Sports Nutr* 14, 33 (2017). https://doi.org/10.1186/s12970-017-0189-4

iv. Thomas DT, Erdman KA, Burke LM. American College of Sports Medicine Joint Position Statement. Nutrition and Athletic Performance. Med Sci Sports Exerc. 2016 Mar;48(3):543-68. doi: 10.1249/MSS.0000000000000852. Erratum in: Med Sci Sports Exerc. 2017 Jan;49(1):222. doi: 10.1249/MSS.0000000000001162. PMID: 26891166.

v. Conz, Andrea et al. "Effect of Non-Nutritive Sweeteners on the Gut Microbiota." *Nutrients* vol. 15,8 1869. 13 Apr. 2023, doi:10.3390/nu15081869

vi. Sweetness Intensity of Sweeteners Compared to Table Sugar . (n.d.). Food and Drug Administration. Retrieved from https://www.fda.gov/media/168345/download.

vii. World Health Organization. (14 July 2023). *Aspartame hazard and risk assess-*

ment results released. World Health Organization. https://www.who.int/news/item/14-07-2023-aspartame-hazard-and-risk-assessment-results-released

3. PROTEIN IS A PRIORITY

i. McLean, C.P., Kulkarni, J. & Sharp, G. Disordered eating and the meat-avoidance spectrum: a systematic review and clinical implications. *Eat Weight Disord* 27, 2347–2375 (2022). https://doi.org/10.1007/s40519-022-01428-0
ii. Jacobs, David R Jr et al. "Food synergy: an operational concept for understanding nutrition." *The American journal of clinical nutrition* vol. 89,5 (2009): 1543S-1548S. doi:10.3945/ajcn.2009.26736B
iii. Bandara SB, Towle KM, Monnot AD. A human health risk assessment of heavy metal ingestion among consumers of protein powder supplements. Toxicol Rep. 2020 Aug 21;7:1255-1262. doi: 10.1016/j.toxrep.2020.08.001. PMID: 33005567; PMCID: PMC7509468.
iv. Kerksick, C.M., Wilborn, C.D., Roberts, M.D. et al. ISSN exercise & sports nutrition review update: research & recommendations. *J Int Soc Sports Nutr* 15, 38 (2018). https://doi.org/10.1186/s12970-018-0242-y
v. *When it comes to protein, how much is too much?*. Harvard Health. (2024, July 23). https://www.health.harvard.edu/nutrition/when-it-comes-to-protein-how-much-is-too-much
vi. Institute of Medicine (US) Committee on Military Nutrition Research. The Role of Protein and Amino Acids in Sustaining and Enhancing Performance. Washington (DC): National Academies Press (US); 1999. 14, Amino Acid and Protein Requirements: Cognitive Performance, Stress, and Brain Function. Available from: https://www.ncbi.nlm.nih.gov/books/NBK224629/

4. FAT IS YOUR FRIEND

i. American Dietetic Association; Dietitians of Canada; American College of Sports Medicine; Rodriguez NR, Di Marco NM, Langley S. American College of Sports Medicine position stand. Nutrition and athletic performance. Med Sci Sports Exerc. 2009 Mar;41(3):709-31. doi: 10.1249/MSS.0b013e31890eb86. PMID: 19225360.
ii. Holtzman B, Ackerman KE. Recommendations and Nutritional Considerations for Female Athletes: Health and Performance. Sports Med. 2021 Sep;51(Suppl 1):43-57. doi: 10.1007/s40279-021-01508-8. Epub 2021 Sep 13. PMID: 34515972; PMCID: PMC8566643.
iii. Burke LM, Kiens B, Ivy JL. Carbohydrates and fat for training and recovery. J Sports Sci. 2004 Jan;22(1):15-30. doi: 10.1080/0264041031000140527. PMID: 14971430.
iv. World Health Organization. (December 7 2021). *Countries with regulations protecting people from industrially produced trans fat tripled over the past year*. World Health Organization. https://www.who.int/news/item/07-12-2021-

      countries-with-regulations-protecting-people-from-industrially-produced-trans-fat-tripled-over-the-past-year

  v. Kerksick, C.M., Wilborn, C.D., Roberts, M.D. et al. ISSN exercise & sports nutrition review update: research & recommendations. J Int Soc Sports Nutr 15, 38 (2018). https://doi.org/10.1186/s12970-018-0242-y

  vi. Tomczyk M, Heileson JL, Babiarz M, Calder PC. Athletes Can Benefit from Increased Intake of EPA and DHA-Evaluating the Evidence. Nutrients. 2023 Nov 26;15(23):4925. doi: 10.3390/nu15234925. PMID: 38068783; PMCID: PMC10708277.

  vii. Dobranowska, K., Plińska, S., & Dobosz, A. (2024). Dietary and Lifestyle Management of Functional Hypothalamic Amenorrhea: A Comprehensive Review. *Nutrients*, 16(17), 2967. https://doi.org/10.3390/nu16172967

5. MICRONUTRIENTS: WHAT ARE THEY + WHY DO THEY MATTER?

  i. Owens DJ, Allison R, Close GL. Vitamin D and the Athlete: Current Perspectives and New Challenges. Sports Med. 2018 Mar;48(Suppl 1):3-16. doi: 10.1007/s40279-017-0841-9. PMID: 29368183; PMCID: PMC5790847.

  ii. Srivastava, Sneha Baxi. "Vitamin D: Do We Need More Than Sunshine?." *American journal of lifestyle medicine* vol. 15,4 397-401. 3 Apr. 2021, doi:10.1177/1559827621100 5689

  iii. Conway, D., & Henderson, M. A. (2019). Iron metabolism. *Anaesthesia & Intensive Care Medicine*, 20(3), 175–177. https://doi.org/10.1016/j.mpaic.2019.01.003

  iv. Sim M, Garvican-Lewis LA, Cox GR, Govus A, McKay AKA, Stellingwerff T, Peeling P. Iron considerations for the athlete: a narrative review. Eur J Appl Physiol. 2019 Jul;119(7):1463-1478. doi: 10.1007/s00421-019-04157-y. Epub 2019 May 4. PMID: 31055680.

  v. Coad J, Conlon C. Iron deficiency in women: assessment, causes and consequences. Curr Opin Clin Nutr Metab Care. 2011 Nov;14(6):625-34. doi: 10.1097/MCO.0b013e32834be6fd. PMID: 21934611.

  vi. Cleveland Clinic. (2025, May 9). *Iron deficiency: An under-recognized condition in female athletes*. https://consultqd.clevelandclinic.org/iron-deficiency-an-under-recognized-condition-in-female-athletes

  vii. U.S. Department of Health and Human Services. (August 13, 2023). *Office of dietary supplements - iron*. NIH Office of Dietary Supplements. https://ods.od.nih.gov/factsheets/Iron-Consumer/

  viii. Office of the Surgeon General (US). Bone Health and Osteoporosis: A Report of the Surgeon General. Rockville (MD): Office of the Surgeon General (US); 2004. 2, The Basics of Bone in Health and Disease. https://www.ncbi.nlm.nih.gov/books/NBK45504/

  ix. Gehman, Sarah et al. "Restrictive Eating and Prior Low-Energy Fractures Are Associated With History of Multiple Bone Stress Injuries." *International journal of sport nutrition and exercise metabolism* vol. 32,5 325-333. 6 May. 2022, doi:10.1123/ijsnem.2021-0323

x. Fensham, Nikita C et al. "Short-Term Carbohydrate Restriction Impairs Bone Formation at Rest and During Prolonged Exercise to a Greater Degree than Low Energy Availability." *Journal of bone and mineral research : the official journal of the American Society for Bone and Mineral Research* vol. 37,10 (2022): 1915-1925. doi:10.1002/jbmr.4658

xi. Roche, Megan et al. "Higher Triad Risk Scores Are Associated With Increased Risk for Trabecular-Rich Bone Stress Injuries in Female Runners." *Clinical journal of sport medicine : official journal of the Canadian Academy of Sport Medicine* vol. 33,6 (2023): 631-637. doi:10.1097/JSM.0000000000001180

xii. Barry, Daniel W et al. "Acute calcium ingestion attenuates exercise-induced disruption of calcium homeostasis." *Medicine and science in sports and exercise* vol. 43,4 (2011): 617-23. doi:10.1249/MSS.0b013e31811f79fa8

xiii. Mountjoy M, Sundgot-Borgen J, Burke L, Carter S, Constantini N, Lebrun C, Meyer N, Sherman R, Steffen K, Budgett R, Ljungqvist A. The IOC consensus statement: beyond the Female Athlete Triad--Relative Energy Deficiency in Sport (RED-S). Br J Sports Med. 2014 Apr;48(7):491-7. doi: 10.1136/bjsports-2014-093502. PMID: 24620037.

xiv. Zhang Y, Xun P, Wang R, Mao L, He K. Can Magnesium Enhance Exercise Performance? Nutrients. 2017 Aug 28;9(9):946. doi: 10.3390/nu9090946. PMID: 28846654; PMCID: PMC5622706.

xv. Krzywański J, Mikulski T, Pokrywka A, Młyńczak M, Krysztofiak H, Frączek B, Ziemba A. Vitamin B12 Status and Optimal Range for Hemoglobin Formation in Elite Athletes. Nutrients. 2020 Apr 9;12(4):1038. doi: 10.3390/nu12041038. PMID: 32283824; PMCID: PMC7230602.

xvi. Niklewicz, Ali et al. "The importance of vitamin B12 for individuals choosing plant-based diets." *European journal of nutrition* vol. 62,3 (2023): 1551-1559. doi:10.1007/s00394-022-03025-4

xvii. Elangovan R and Baruteau J (2022) Inherited and acquired vitamin B12 deficiencies: Which administration route to choose for supplementation?. *Front. Pharmacol.* 13:972468. doi: 10.3389/fphar.2022.972468

xviii. Harvard University. (2024, November 7). *Salt and sodium.* The Nutrition Source. https://nutritionsource.hsph.harvard.edu/salt-and-sodium/

xix. U.S. Food and Drug Administration (March 5, 2024). *Sodium in your diet.* U.S. Food and Drug Administration. https://www.fda.gov/food/nutrition-education-resources-materials/sodium-your-diet

xx. Pérez-Castillo, Íñigo M et al. "Compositional Aspects of Beverages Designed to Promote Hydration Before, During, and After Exercise: Concepts Revisited." *Nutrients* vol. 16,1 17. 20 Dec. 2023, doi:10.3390/nu16010017

xxi. Hew-Butler T. Exercise-Associated Hyponatremia. Front Horm Res. 2019;52:178-189. doi: 10.1159/000493247. Epub 2019 Jan 15. PMID: 32097926.

xxii. American College of Sports Medicine; Sawka MN, Burke LM, Eichner ER, Maughan RJ, Montain SJ, Stachenfeld NS. American College of Sports Medicine position stand. Exercise and fluid replacement. Med Sci Sports Exerc. 2007 Feb;39(2):377-90. doi: 10.1249/mss.0b013e31802ca597. PMID: 17277604.

6. THE PERFORMANCE PLATE

i. Mayo Clinic Health System. (2024, July 25). *Processed Foods: What you should know*. Mayo Clinic Health System. https://www.mayoclinichealthsystem.org/hometown-health/speaking-of-health/processed-foods-what-you-should-know

ii. Eck, Kaitlyn M, and Carol Byrd-Bredbenner. "Food Choice Decisions of Collegiate Division I Athletes: A Qualitative Exploratory Study." *Nutrients* vol. 13,7 2322. 6 Jul. 2021, doi:10.3390/nu13072322

7. PRE-WORKOUT FUELING

i. Rehrer, N J et al. "Gastrointestinal complaints in relation to dietary intake in triathletes." *International journal of sport nutrition* vol. 2,1 (1992): 48-59. doi:10.1123/ijsn.2.1.48

ii. Thomas, D Travis et al. "American College of Sports Medicine Joint Position Statement. Nutrition and Athletic Performance." Medicine and science in sports and exercise vol. 48,3 (2016): 543-68. doi:10.1249/MSS.0000000000000852

iii. Thomas DT, Erdman KA, Burke LM. American College of Sports Medicine Joint Position Statement. Nutrition and Athletic Performance. Med Sci Sports Exerc. 2016 Mar;48(3):543-68. doi: 10.1249/MSS.0000000000000852. Erratum in: Med Sci Sports Exerc. 2017 Jan;49(1):222. doi: 10.1249/MSS.0000000000001162. PMID: 26891166.

iv. Gutiérrez-Hellín, Jorge, and David Varillas-Delgado. "Energy Drinks and Sports Performance, Cardiovascular Risk, and Genetic Associations; Future Prospects." *Nutrients* vol. 13,3 715. 24 Feb. 2021, doi:10.3390/nu13030715

v. Reddy, V. S., Shiva, S., Manikantan, S., & Ramakrishna, S. (2024). Pharmacology of caffeine and its effects on the human body. European Journal of Medicinal Chemistry Reports, 10, 100138. https://doi.org/10.1016/j.ejmcr.2024.100138

vi. *NCAA banned substances*. NCAA.org. (2015, June 10). https://www.ncaa.org/sports/2015/6/10/ncaa-banned-substances.aspx

8. DURING TRAINING + COMPETITION

i. Vitale, Kenneth, and Andrew Getzin. "Nutrition and Supplement Update for the Endurance Athlete: Review and Recommendations." *Nutrients* vol. 11,6 1289. 7 Jun. 2019, doi:10.3390/nu11061289

ii. Murray, Bob, and Christine Rosenbloom. "Fundamentals of glycogen metabolism for coaches and athletes." *Nutrition reviews* vol. 76,4 (2018): 243-259. doi:10.1093/nutrit/nuy001

iii. Currell, Kevin, and Asker E Jeukendrup. "Superior endurance performance with ingestion of multiple transportable carbohydrates." *Medicine and science*

      in sports and exercise vol. 40,2 (2008): 275-81. doi:10.1249/mss.0b013e31815adf19
- iv. Baker, Lindsay B. "Sweating Rate and Sweat Sodium Concentration in Athletes: A Review of Methodology and Intra/Interindividual Variability." *Sports medicine (Auckland, N.Z.)* vol. 47,Suppl 1 (2017): 111-128. doi:10.1007/s40279-017-0691-5
- v. Veniamakis, Eleftherios et al. "Effects of Sodium Intake on Health and Performance in Endurance and Ultra-Endurance Sports." *International journal of environmental research and public health* vol. 19,6 3651. 19 Mar. 2022, doi:10.3390/ijerph19063651
- vi. Buck E, McAllister R, Schroeder JD. Exercise-Associated Hyponatremia. [Updated 2023 Jun 12]. In: StatPearls [Internet]. Treasure Island (FL): StatPearls Publishing; 2025 Jan-. Available from: https://www.ncbi.nlm.nih.gov/books/NBK572128/
- vii. Cheuvront, Samuel N, and Robert W Kenefick. "Dehydration: physiology, assessment, and performance effects." *Comprehensive Physiology* vol. 4,1 (2014): 257-85. doi:10.1002/cphy.c130017
- viii. Veniamakis, Eleftherios et al. "Effects of Sodium Intake on Health and Performance in Endurance and Ultra-Endurance Sports." *International journal of environmental research and public health* vol. 19,6 3651. 19 Mar. 2022, doi:10.3390/ijerph19063651
- ix. Shirreffs, Susan M, and Michael N Sawka. "Fluid and electrolyte needs for training, competition, and recovery." *Journal of sports sciences* vol. 29 Suppl 1 (2011): S39-46. doi:10.1080/02640414.2011.614269
- x. American College of Sports Medicine et al. "American College of Sports Medicine position stand. Exercise and fluid replacement." *Medicine and science in sports and exercise* vol. 39,2 (2007): 377-90. doi:10.1249/mss.0b013e31802ca597
- xi. Naderi, Alireza et al. "Carbohydrates and Endurance Exercise: A Narrative Review of a Food First Approach." *Nutrients* vol. 15,6 1367. 11 Mar. 2023, doi:10.3390/nu15061367
- xii. Naderi, Alireza et al. "Carbohydrates and Endurance Exercise: A Narrative Review of a Food First Approach." *Nutrients* vol. 15,6 1367. 11 Mar. 2023, doi:10.3390/nu15061367

9. POST-WORKOUT FUELING

- i. Kerksick, Chad et al. "International Society of Sports Nutrition position stand: nutrient timing." *Journal of the International Society of Sports Nutrition* vol. 5 17. 3 Oct. 2008, doi:10.1186/1550-2783-5-17

10. COMMON DIGESTIVE ISSUES

- i. Pugh, Jamie N et al. "More than a gut feeling: What is the role of the gastroin-

testinal tract in female athlete health?." *European journal of sport science* vol. 22,5 (2022): 755-764. doi:10.1080/17461391.2021.1921853
ii. Diduch, Barry Kent. "Gastrointestinal Conditions in the Female Athlete." *Clinics in sports medicine* vol. 36,4 (2017): 655-669. doi:10.1016/j.csm.2017.06.001
iii. Shokouhi, Nasim et al. "Development of a new version of the Bristol Stool Form Scale: translation, content validity, face validity, and reliability of the Persian version." *BMJ open gastroenterology* vol. 9,1 (2022): e001017. doi:10.1136/bmjgast-2022-001017
iv. Heaton, K W et al. "Defecation frequency and timing, and stool form in the general population: a prospective study." *Gut* vol. 33,6 (1992): 818-24. doi:10.1136/gut.33.6.818
v. Pugh, Jamie N et al. "More than a gut feeling: What is the role of the gastrointestinal tract in female athlete health?." *European journal of sport science* vol. 22,5 (2022): 755-764. doi:10.1080/17461391.2021.1921853
vi. Norris, Mark L et al. "Gastrointestinal complications associated with anorexia nervosa: A systematic review." *The International journal of eating disorders* vol. 49,3 (2016): 216-37. doi:10.1002/eat.22462
vii. Santonicola, Antonella et al. "Eating Disorders and Gastrointestinal Diseases." *Nutrients* vol. 11,12 3038. 12 Dec. 2019, doi:10.3390/nu11123038
viii. O'Brien, Marcus T et al. "The Athlete Gut Microbiome and its Relevance to Health and Performance: A Review." *Sports medicine (Auckland, N.Z.)* vol. 52,Suppl 1 (2022): 119-128. doi:10.1007/s40279-022-01785-x
ix. Ackerman, Kathryn E et al. "Low energy availability surrogates correlate with health and performance consequences of Relative Energy Deficiency in Sport." *British journal of sports medicine* vol. 53,10 (2019): 628-633. doi:10.1136/bjsports-2017-098958
x. Allaband, Celeste et al. "Microbiome 101: Studying, Analyzing, and Interpreting Gut Microbiome Data for Clinicians." *Clinical gastroenterology and hepatology : the official clinical practice journal of the American Gastroenterological Association* vol. 17,2 (2019): 218-230. doi:10.1016/j.cgh.2018.09.017
xi. Thackray, A. E., & Stensel, D. J. (2023). The impact of acute exercise on appetite control: Current insights and future perspectives. *Appetite, 186*, 106557. https://doi.org/10.1016/j.appet.2023.106557
xii. Trexler, Eric T et al. "Metabolic adaptation to weight loss: implications for the athlete." *Journal of the International Society of Sports Nutrition* vol. 11,1 7. 27 Feb. 2014, doi:10.1186/1550-2783-11-7
xiii. Thackray, A. E., & Stensel, D. J. (2023). The impact of acute exercise on appetite control: Current insights and future perspectives. Appetite, 186, 106557. https://doi.org/10.1016/j.appet.2023.106557

11. SLEEP 101

i. Coel, R. A., Pujalte, G. G. A., Applewhite, A. I., Zaslow, T., Cooper, G., Ton, A. N., & Benjamin, H. J. (2022). Sleep and the young athlete. *Sports Health: A*

  Multidisciplinary Approach, 15(4), 537–546. https://doi.org/10.1177/19417381221108732
ii. Schwartz, J., & Simon, R. D. (2015). Sleep extension improves serving accuracy: A study with College Varsity Tennis Players. *Physiology & Behavior, 151*, 541–544. https://doi.org/10.1016/j.physbeh.2015.08.035
iii. Lastella M, Halson SL, Vitale JA, Memon AR, Vincent GE. To Nap or Not to Nap? A Systematic Review Evaluating Napping Behavior in Athletes and the Impact on Various Measures of Athletic Performance. Nat Sci Sleep. 2021 Jun 24;13:841-862. doi: 10.2147/NSS.S315556. PMID: 34194254; PMCID: PMC8238550.

12. UNDERSTAND YOUR HORMONES

i. Cleveland Clinic. (2025, April 4). *Estrogen: Hormone, function, Levels & Imbalances.* Cleveland Clinic. https://my.clevelandclinic.org/health/body/22353-estrogen
ii. Cable JK, Grider MH. Physiology, Progesterone. [Updated 2023 May 1]. In: StatPearls [Internet]. Treasure Island (FL): StatPearls Publishing; 2025 Jan-. Available from: https://www.ncbi.nlm.nih.gov/books/NBK558960/
iii. Mazer, Norman A. "Testosterone deficiency in women: etiologies, diagnosis, and emerging treatments." *International journal of fertility and women's medicine* vol. 47,2 (2002): 77-86.
iv. Southmayd EA, Mallinson RJ, Williams NI, Mallinson DJ, De Souza MJ. Unique effects of energy versus estrogen deficiency on multiple components of bone strength in exercising women. Osteoporos Int. 2017 Apr;28(4):1365-1376. doi: 10.1007/s00198-016-3887-x. Epub 2016 Dec 28. PMID: 28032184.
v. Coelho, Alexandra Ruivo et al. "The Female Athlete Triad/Relative Energy Deficiency in Sports (RED-S)." "A tríade da atleta feminina/déficit energético relativo no esporte (RED-S)." *Revista brasileira de ginecologia e obstetricia : revista da Federacao Brasileira das Sociedades de Ginecologia e Obstetricia* vol. 43,5 (2021): 395-402. doi:10.1055/s-0041-1730289
vi. Heikura IA, Uusitalo ALT, Stellingwerff T, Bergland D, Mero AA, Burke LM. Low Energy Availability Is Difficult to Assess but Outcomes Have Large Impact on Bone Injury Rates in Elite Distance Athletes. Int J Sport Nutr Exerc Metab. 2018 Jul 1;28(4):403-411. doi: 10.1123/ijsnem.2017-0313. Epub 2018 Jun 12. PMID: 29252050.
vii. Cabre HE, Moore SR, Smith-Ryan AE, Hackney AC. Relative Energy Deficiency in Sport (RED-S): Scientific, Clinical, and Practical Implications for the Female Athlete. Dtsch Z Sportmed. 2022;73(7):225-234. doi: 10.5960/dzsm.2022.546. Epub 2022 Nov 1. PMID: 36479178; PMCID: PMC9724109.
viii. Cabre HE, Moore SR, Smith-Ryan AE, Hackney AC. Relative Energy Deficiency in Sport (RED-S): Scientific, Clinical, and Practical Implications for the Female Athlete. Dtsch Z Sportmed. 2022;73(7):225-234. doi:

ix. Stubblefield, P G. "Menstrual impact of contraception." *American journal of obstetrics and gynecology* vol. 170,5 Pt 2 (1994): 1513-22. doi:10.1016/s0002-9378(94)05013-1
x. https://pubmed.ncbi.nlm.nih.gov/23852908/
xi. Pinheiro, Andréa Poyastro et al. "Sexual functioning in women with eating disorders." *The International journal of eating disorders* vol. 43,2 (2010): 123-9. doi:10.1002/eat.20671
xii. Colenso-Semple LM, D'Souza AC, Elliott-Sale KJ, Phillips SM. Current evidence shows no influence of women's menstrual cycle phase on acute strength performance or adaptations to resistance exercise training. Front Sports Act Living. 2023 Mar 23;5:1054542. doi: 10.3389/fspor.2023.1054542. PMID: 37033884; PMCID: PMC10076834.

McNulty KL, Elliott-Sale KJ, Dolan E, Swinton PA, Ansdell P, Goodall S, Thomas K, Hicks KM. The Effects of Menstrual Cycle Phase on Exercise Performance in Eumenorrheic Women: A Systematic Review and Meta-Analysis. Sports Med. 2020 Oct;50(10):1813-1827. doi: 10.1007/s40279-020-01319-3. PMID: 32661839; PMCID: PMC7497427.
xiii. Carmichael, Mikaeli Anne et al. "The Impact of Menstrual Cycle Phase on Athletes' Performance: A Narrative Review." *International journal of environmental research and public health* vol. 18,4 1667. 9 Feb. 2021, doi:10.3390/ijerph18041667
xiv. McNulty, Kelly Lee et al. "The Effects of Menstrual Cycle Phase on Exercise Performance in Eumenorrheic Women: A Systematic Review and Meta-Analysis." *Sports medicine (Auckland, N.Z.)* vol. 50,10 (2020): 1813-1827. doi:10.1007/s40279-020-01319-3
xv. Logue, Danielle M et al. "Low Energy Availability in Athletes 2020: An Updated Narrative Review of Prevalence, Risk, Within-Day Energy Balance, Knowledge, and Impact on Sports Performance." *Nutrients* vol. 12,3 835. 20 Mar. 2020, doi:10.3390/nu12030835

13. WHAT HAPPENS WHEN YOU UNDERFUEL?

i. Mountjoy M, Ackerman KE, Bailey DM, Burke LM, Constantini N, Hackney AC, Heikura IA, Melin A, Pensgaard AM, Stellingwerff T, Sundgot-Borgen JK, Torstveit MK, Jacobsen AU, Verhagen E, Budgett R, Engebretsen L, Erdener U. 2023 International Olympic Committee's (IOC) consensus statement on Relative Energy Deficiency in Sport (REDs). Br J Sports Med. 2023 Sep;57(17):1073-1097. doi: 10.1136/bjsports-2023-106994. Erratum in: Br J Sports Med. 2024 Feb 7;58(3):e4. doi: 10.1136/bjsports-2023-106994corr1. PMID: 37752011.
ii. Stellingwerff, Trent et al. "Overtraining Syndrome (OTS) and Relative Energy Deficiency in Sport (RED-S): Shared Pathways, Symptoms and Complexities." *Sports medicine (Auckland, N.Z.)* vol. 51,11 (2021): 2251-2280. doi:10.1007/s40279-021-01491-0

iii. Jeppesen, Jan S et al. "Short-Term Severe Low Energy Availability in Athletes: Molecular Mechanisms, Endocrine Responses, and Performance Outcomes A Narrative Review." *Scandinavian journal of medicine & science in sports* vol. 35,6 (2025): e70089. doi:10.1111/sms.70089

iv. Stellingwerff, Trent et al. "Review of the scientific rationale, development and validation of the International Olympic Committee Relative Energy Deficiency in Sport Clinical Assessment Tool: V.2 (IOC REDs CAT2)-by a subgroup of the IOC consensus on REDs." *British journal of sports medicine* vol. 57,17 (2023): 1109-1118. doi:10.1136/bjsports-2023-106914

v. Sale C, Elliott-Sale KJ. Nutrition and Athlete Bone Health. Sports Med. 2019 Dec;49(Suppl 2):139-151. doi: 10.1007/s40279-019-01161-2. PMID: 31696454; PMCID: PMC6901417.

vi. Fensham NC, Heikura IA, McKay AKA, Tee N, Ackerman KE, Burke LM. Short-Term Carbohydrate Restriction Impairs Bone Formation at Rest and During Prolonged Exercise to a Greater Degree than Low Energy Availability. J Bone Miner Res. 2022 Oct;37(10):1915-1925. doi: 10.1002/jbmr.4658. Epub 2022 Aug 10. PMID: 35869933; PMCID: PMC9804216.

vii. Melin AK, Heikura IA, Tenforde A, Mountjoy M. Energy Availability in Athletics: Health, Performance, and Physique. Int J Sport Nutr Exerc Metab. 2019 Mar 1;29(2):152-164. doi: 10.1123/ijsnem.2018-0201. Epub 2019 Feb 26. PMID: 30632422.

viii. Saadedine, Mariam et al. "Functional Hypothalamic Amenorrhea: Recognition and Management of a Challenging Diagnosis." *Mayo Clinic proceedings* vol. 98,9 (2023): 1376-1385. doi:10.1016/j.mayocp.2023.05.027

ix. Pensgaard AM, Sundgot-Borgen J, Edwards C, *et al* Intersection of mental health issues and Relative Energy Deficiency in Sport (REDs): a narrative review by a subgroup of the IOC consensus on REDs *British Journal of Sports Medicine* 2023;57:1127-1135.

x. Torres-McGehee, Toni M et al. "Energy Availability With or Without Eating Disorder Risk in Collegiate Female Athletes and Performing Artists." *Journal of athletic training* vol. 56,9 (2021): 993-1002. doi:10.4085/JAT0502-20

xi. Sundgot-Borgen C, Sundgot-Borgen J, Sølvberg N, *et al* Factors predicting disordered eating and the prevalence of eating disorders in adolescent elite athletes, trained athletes and a reference group: a prospective controlled two-step study *British Journal of Sports Medicine* Published Online First: 17 March 2025. doi: 10.1136/bjsports-2024-108808

xii. Klungland Torstveit, Monica, and Jorunn Sundgot-Borgen. "Are under- and overweight female elite athletes thin and fat? A controlled study." *Medicine and science in sports and exercise* vol. 44,5 (2012): 949-57. doi:10.1249/MSS.0b013e31823fe4ef

xiii. *Project Red-S: A RED-s recovery game plan.* Project RED-s. (n.d.). https://red-s.com/articles/your-reds-recovery-game-plan

xiv. Klungland Torstveit, Monica, and Jorunn Sundgot-Borgen. "Are under- and overweight female elite athletes thin and fat? A controlled study." *Medicine and science in sports and exercise* vol. 44,5 (2012): 949-57. doi:10.1249/MSS.0b013e31823fe4ef

xv. Marzuki MIH, Mohamad MI, Chai WJ, Farah NMF, Safii NS, Jasme JK, Jamil NA. Prevalence of Relative Energy Deficiency in Sport (RED-S) among National Athletes in Malaysia. Nutrients. 2023 Mar 30;15(7):1697. doi: 10.3390/nu15071697. PMID: 37049534; PMCID: PMC10096906.

xvi. Hicks, L. (2020, July 29). *For young female athletes, losing weight may not improve performance* American Association for the Advancement of Science - Science.org. doi: 10.1126/science.abe0757

xvii. Uchizawa, Akiko et al. "Differential Risks of the Duration and Degree of Weight Control on Bone Health and Menstruation in Female Athletes." *Frontiers in nutrition* vol. 9 875802. 26 Apr. 2022, doi:10.3389/fnut.2022.875802

xviii. Li, Qingqing et al. "Athlete Body Image and Eating Disorders: A Systematic Review of Their Association and Influencing Factors." *Nutrients* vol. 16,16 2686. 13 Aug. 2024, doi:10.3390/nu16162686

xix. Torres-McGehee, Toni M et al. "Sports nutrition knowledge among collegiate athletes, coaches, athletic trainers, and strength and conditioning specialists." *Journal of athletic training* vol. 47,2 (2012): 205-11. doi:10.4085/1062-6050-47.2.205

14. WHAT'S THE DEAL WITH SUPPLEMENTS?

i. Mathews, Neilson M. "Prohibited Contaminants in Dietary Supplements." *Sports health* vol. 10,1 (2018): 19-30. doi:10.1177/1941738117727736

ii. U.S. Anti-Doping Agency (USADA). (2023, July 5). *Third-party testing guidance.* U.S. Anti-Doping Agency (USADA). https://www.usada.org/athletes/substances/supplement-connect/reduce-risk-testing-positive-experiencing-adverse-health-effects/third-party-testing-guidance/

iii. Hurrell, Richard, and Ines Egli. "Iron bioavailability and dietary reference values." *The American journal of clinical nutrition* vol. 91,5 (2010): 1461S-1467S. doi:10.3945/ajcn.2010.28674F

iv. Badenhorst, Claire E et al. "Iron status in athletic females, a shift in perspective on an old paradigm." *Journal of sports sciences* vol. 39,14 (2021): 1565-1575. doi:10.1080/02640414.2021.1885782

v. Papanikolaou, G, and K Pantopoulos. "Iron metabolism and toxicity." *Toxicology and applied pharmacology* vol. 202,2 (2005): 199-211. doi:10.1016/j.taap.2004.06.021

vi. Sim, Marc et al. "Iron considerations for the athlete: a narrative review." *European journal of applied physiology* vol. 119,7 (2019): 1463-1478. doi:10.1007/s00421-019-04157-y

vii. Wasserfurth, Paulina et al. "Reasons for and Consequences of Low Energy Availability in Female and Male Athletes: Social Environment, Adaptations, and Prevention." *Sports medicine - open* vol. 6,1 44. 10 Sep. 2020, doi:10.1186/s40798-020-00275-6

viii. Wasserfurth, Paulina et al. "Reasons for and Consequences of Low Energy Availability in Female and Male Athletes: Social Environment, Adaptations,

ix. and Prevention." *Sports medicine - open* vol. 6,1 44. 10 Sep. 2020, doi:10.1186/s40798-020-00275-6

ix. Newlin, Mia K et al. "The effects of acute exercise bouts on hepcidin in women." *International journal of sport nutrition and exercise metabolism* vol. 22,2 (2012): 79-88. doi:10.1123/ijsnem.22.2.79

x. McCormick, Rachel et al. "The Impact of Morning versus Afternoon Exercise on Iron Absorption in Athletes." *Medicine and science in sports and exercise* vol. 51,10 (2019): 2147-2155. doi:10.1249/MSS.0000000000002026

xi. Yuen, H.-W. (2023, June 26). *Iron toxicity*. U.S. National Library of Medicine. https://www.ncbi.nlm.nih.gov/books/NBK459224/

xii. *NCAA banned substances*. NCAA.org. (2015, June 10). https://www.ncaa.org/sports/2015/6/10/ncaa-banned-substances.aspx

xiii. Cappelletti, Simone et al. "Caffeine-Related Deaths: Manner of Deaths and Categories at Risk." *Nutrients* vol. 10,5 611. 14 May. 2018, doi:10.3390/nu10050611

xiv. Barretto, Junaura Rocha et al. "Use of dietary supplements by children and adolescents." *Jornal de pediatria* vol. 100 Suppl 1,Suppl 1 (2024): S31-S39. doi:10.1016/j.jped.2023.09.008

xv. Dwyer, Johanna T et al. "Do Multivitamin/Mineral Dietary Supplements for Young Children Fill Critical Nutrient Gaps?." *Journal of the Academy of Nutrition and Dietetics* vol. 122,3 (2022): 525-532. doi:10.1016/j.jand.2021.10.019

xvi. Anderson, Nash et al. "Under-representation of women is alive and well in sport and exercise medicine: what it looks like and what we can do about it." *BMJ open sport & exercise medicine* vol. 9,2 e001606. 5 Apr. 2023, doi:10.1136/bmjsem-2023-001606

15. WHAT NUTRITION TRENDS GET WRONG

i. Blumberg, Jack et al. "Intermittent fasting: consider the risks of disordered eating for your patient." *Clinical diabetes and endocrinology* vol. 9,1 4. 21 Oct. 2023, doi:10.1186/s40842-023-00152-7

ii. Ahokas, Essi K et al. "A post-exercise infrared sauna session improves recovery of neuromuscular performance and muscle soreness after resistance exercise training." *Biology of sport* vol. 40,3 (2023): 681-689. doi:10.5114/biolsport.2023.119289

iii. Ahokas, Essi K et al. "A post-exercise infrared sauna session improves recovery of neuromuscular performance and muscle soreness after resistance exercise training." *Biology of sport* vol. 40,3 (2023): 681-689. doi:10.5114/biolsport.2023.119289

iv. Malone, Jordan C. and Sharon F. Daley. "Elimination Diets." *StatPearls*, StatPearls Publishing, 9 January 2024.

v. Myrissa, K., Jackson, L., & Kelaiditi, E. (2023). Orthorexia nervosa: Examining the reliability and validity of two self-report measures and the predictors of orthorexic symptoms in elite and recreational athletes. *Performance Enhancement & Health*, 11(4), 100265. https://doi.org/10.1016/j.peh.2023.100265

vi. Tchounwou, Paul B et al. "Heavy metal toxicity and the environment." *Experientia supplementum* (2012) vol. 101 (2012): 133-64. doi:10.1007/978-3-7643-8340-4_6

vii. Cross, J. (2001). Megacities and small towns: Different perspectives on hazard vulnerability. *Global Environmental Change Part B: Environmental Hazards*, 3(2), 63–80. https://doi.org/10.1016/s1464-2867(01)00020-1

viii. Environmental Protection Agency. (2025, May 22). *Basic Information about Lead in Drinking Water*. Environmental Protection Agency. https://www.epa.gov/ground-water-and-drinking-water/basic-information-about-lead-drinking-water

ix. *Dietary supplements linked with severe health events in children, young adults*. Harvard T.H. Chan School of Public Health. (2024, November 22). https://hsph.harvard.edu/news/dietary-supplements-health-risks-youth/

x. Allaband, Celeste et al. "Microbiome 101: Studying, Analyzing, and Interpreting Gut Microbiome Data for Clinicians." *Clinical gastroenterology and hepatology : the official clinical practice journal of the American Gastroenterological Association* vol. 17,2 (2019): 218-230. doi:10.1016/j.cgh.2018.09.017

xi. Navarro, Victor J et al. "Liver injury from herbal and dietary supplements." *Hepatology (Baltimore, Md.)* vol. 65,1 (2017): 363-373. doi:10.1002/hep.28813

xii. Cienfuegos, Sofia et al. "Effect of Intermittent Fasting on Reproductive Hormone Levels in Females and Males: A Review of Human Trials." *Nutrients* vol. 14,11 2343. 3 Jun. 2022, doi:10.3390/nu14112343

xiii. Harvie, Michelle, and Mai Haiba. "The impact of intermittent energy restriction on women's health." *The Proceedings of the Nutrition Society*, 1-10. 11 Feb. 2025, doi:10.1017/S0029665125000059

xiv. Lacy, Brian E et al. "Leaky Gut Syndrome: Myths and Management." *Gastroenterology & hepatology* vol. 20,5 (2024): 264-272.

xv. Lacy, Brian E et al. "Leaky Gut Syndrome: Myths and Management." *Gastroenterology & hepatology* vol. 20,5 (2024): 264-272.

xvi. Bischoff, Stephan C et al. "Intestinal permeability--a new target for disease prevention and therapy." *BMC gastroenterology* vol. 14 189. 18 Nov. 2014, doi:10.1186/s12876-014-0189-7

xvii. *Therapeutic use exemptions (tues)*. World Anti Doping Agency. (2024, June 11). https://www.wada-ama.org/en/athletes-support-personnel/therapeutic-use-exemptions-tues

xviii. *Intravenous infusions and/or injections*. World Anti-Doping Agency. (2018, January 1). https://www.wada-ama.org/sites/default/files/resources/files/intravenous_infusions_v5.0_jan2018_en.pdf

xix. Furman, David et al. "Chronic inflammation in the etiology of disease across the life span." *Nature medicine* vol. 25,12 (2019): 1822-1832. doi:10.1038/s41591-019-0675-0

xx. Dinetz, Elliot, and Nataliya Bocharova. "Inflammation in Elite Athletes: A Review of Novel Factors, the Role of Microbiome, and Treatments for Performance Longevity." *Cureus* vol. 16,10 e72720. 30 Oct. 2024, doi:10.7759/cureus.72720

xxi. Tipton, Kevin D. "Nutritional Support for Exercise-Induced Injuries." *Sports medicine (Auckland, N.Z.)* vol. 45 Suppl 1 (2015): S93-104. doi:10.1007/s40279-015-0398-4

22. HOW TO TALK TO EXPERTS—AND BE TAKEN SERIOUSLY

i. TodayShow. (2019, May 17). *Feel discriminated against at the Doctor's Office? you're not alone.* TODAY.com. https://www.today.com/health/today-survey-finds-gender-discrimination-doctor-s-office-serious-issue-t153641
ii. Johns, C. (2019, June 13). *The diagnosis of exclusion.* PM Pediatric Care. https://pmpediatriccare.com/blog/the-diagnosis-of-exclusion/
iii. Kim, Young Sun, and Nayoung Kim. "Sex-Gender Differences in Irritable Bowel Syndrome." *Journal of neurogastroenterology and motility* vol. 24,4 (2018): 544-558. doi:10.5056/jnm18082
iv. McLean, Carmen P et al. "Gender differences in anxiety disorders: prevalence, course of illness, comorbidity and burden of illness." *Journal of psychiatric research* vol. 45,8 (2011): 1027-35. doi:10.1016/j.jpsychires.2011.03.006
v. Tai-Seale, Ming et al. "Time allocation in primary care office visits." *Health services research* vol. 42,5 (2007): 1871-94. doi:10.1111/j.1475-6773.2006.00689.x

26 / MORE FROM STRONG GIRL PUBLISHING

Shred Girls Series

Lindsay's Joyride
Ali's Rocky Ride
Jen's Bumpy Ride
Lindsay and the Curse of Gemini Lakes

Other Titles from Strong Girl Publishing

The Mirror Diaries: Finding Grace by Vanessa Coulbeck
The Strong Girl by Molly Hurford
In Defense of Big Dreams by Mackenzie Myatt
Running as Fast as We Can by Molly Hurford
Sprinting Through Setbacks by Micha Powell
Best Day Ever Journal by Rachel Pageau
The Athlete's Guide to Sponsorship by Molly Hurford

FIND MORE books like this at StrongGirlPublishing.com

www.ingramcontent.com/pod-product-compliance
Lightning Source LLC
Chambersburg PA
CBHW051545020426
42333CB00016B/2099